BEYOND DIETING

An Edgar Cayce Program for Permanent Weight Control

by Linda Cochran

A.R.E.® PRESS • VIRGINIA BEACH • VIRGINIA

Note to the reader:
Most of the selections from the Edgar Cayce readings appear in boldface type. The number following each reading is the file number assigned to the person or group for whom the reading was given. For example, 317-6 identifies the sixth reading given for the person who was assigned number 317.

All Cayce readings (over 14,000) are available for public inspection at the A.R.E. Library in Virginia Beach, Virginia.

Printed in the U.S.A.

The Seven Levels

This book is dedicated to everyone who understands that successful people are manifestations of their imaginations.

Introduction

I wanted to title this book *Remodel the Temple*, but we've heard so often in metaphysical circles "the body is the temple of God" that it has become a cliché.

The purpose of this book is to show that application to the physical body of the principles found in *A Search for God*, Books I & II,* can lead to internal revelations that may produce external transformations, and, hence, a remodeling of the temple.

Not written for the masses, this book contains certain presumptions about its readers: (1) that they are familiar with Edgar Cayce; (2) that they know about A.R.E. Study Groups; (3) that they know that A.R.E. stands for "Always Ready to Eat," as well as Association for Research and Enlightenment; and (4) that they have a sense of humor.

Members of Study Groups, in particular, will recognize some expressions more readily than will those who have not experienced being a member of such a Group. If such "inside" terminology tends to cause others to feel left out—good. Maybe they will become curious about what they are missing and will actually read the last page to see how to find a Group nearest them.

Should this book fall into the hands of the "uninitiated," the author disclaims any responsibility for the upheavals in the earth that may occur.

Warning: Should one become interested in the two small slim volumes, entitled *A Search for God*, on which this work is based, it should be noted that referring to these as "the little red books" is tantamount to calling Harvard University the little red schoolhouse.

---

*A Search for God, Books I & II, A.R.E. Press, Virginia Beach, Va., 1942 and 1950.

"This day is set before thee carrots and cake. . . Choose thou."

Level One

"I Can't Do It"

"I can't lose weight because. . ."

Finish that sentence any way you like, and I'll tell you why you are kidding yourself.

I'm not saying it will be easy. What worthwhile thing is?

As a weight-control columnist, I have received letters from readers who were using excuses for not losing weight. Most of their excuses I had used on myself when I had more than 100 pounds to lose.

Two favorites: "I can't lose weight because my thyroid is underactive." "I can't lose weight because I have to cook for my family."

My thyroid was underactive, but as a student of the Edgar Cayce readings I learned that persistent, consistent meditation can regulate the endocrine system—eventually. And while these writings are not intended to teach you how to meditate—you probably already know how—I do hope to show that *acting* on what you know about meditation, prayer, reveries, visualization, journal writing, dreams, ideals, goals, attitudes, emotions, life influences (past and present), self-image building, choices (especially food choices), and exercise does work. It worked for me, and if I can do it, anybody can.

I, too, had to cook for a family, a husband and three sons. They were accustomed to bountiful meals—on time. And when I decided that all that weight had to go, they didn't always get them. But nobody died. In fact, now every one of them is healthier—and slimmer—than they would have been had I not changed my thinking and way of cooking.

You may be, as I was, cooking the wrong foods for your family. If you secretly don't like your husband, overfeeding him is a good way to do him in. And shoving a cookie into a whimpering child's hands establishes deadly patterns for adult life.

Those patterns may have been established in you by your parents and, indeed, you cannot lose weight unless you change them. But you *can* change if you want to. Later, we will look at *if* you want to change. Some don't. But for now let's assume that you do, but you feel that you need your family's cooperation. For me it took courage.

It wasn't easy to stop buying junk food, especially the ones I found irresistible—which included everything. The boys thought they'd starve to death before they learned to eat fruit instead of cookies. And my youngest son had a hard time explaining to his music teacher that he couldn't participate in the fund-raising candy sale "because my mother won't let me bring it in the house."

I would not and will not allow any food into the house that has sugar in it. Along with inheriting a slow metabolism, I chose a grandfather who was blinded with diabetes before he died. Like all prediabetics I am allergic to sugar, which means if I start eating it, I can't stop. Even knowing this about myself does not stop me from craving sugar-laden foods when they are in the house, and who wants to waste all that energy resisting temptation under one's own roof! But try explaining that to a pie-baking grandmother.

My husband's mother bakes pecan pies that are famous in four states. Like any dutiful grandmother, she just adores baking pies for her grandchildren and bringing them over "just in case they should want something sweet." After all, the poor little darlings never get anything special from their mother. Gently I tried explaining, "Mom, I really do appreciate your thinking of the kids, but I wish you would understand that leaving those pies here is like waving a bottle under the nose of an alcoholic."

So when I saw that I wasn't getting anywhere by talking, the next time the pies appeared, I threw them in the lake. Mom nearly collapsed. But better the ducks and turtles get diabetes than me.

Drastic action, sure, but it worked.

Almost as drastic was the first time I refused to cook dinner. In the beginning, before my family's tastes in food changed, they wanted fried chicken and gravy with mashed potatoes for supper. Now, of course, everyone has learned to appreciate beautiful, fresh, live, lightly steamed vegetables, broiled fish or chicken, and fresh fruit—which makes my life so much easier because we all eat the same foods. But before I learned to cook creatively, I was trying to serve them the foods to which they were accustomed, and I spend a lot of time hungry. Learning how to lose weight while never being hungry was an evolutionary process, which I'll tell you about later. So it wasn't easy to look up at my 6'5" husband and say, "I'm not cooking tonight; I'm just too hungry; if I cook, I'll eat, and I'm not going to do that"; then turn around, go to my room, and close the door.

Husbands tend to go into cardiac arrest at such pronouncements, especially when they've seen you fail time after time at losing weight. It can be difficult for them to accept interruptions in their own lives when they believe your efforts are just another temporary attempt at "dieting." So you must be convinced at the rightness and unselfishness of your efforts to continue at these times—which you *will* be after completing the written exercises on the following pages.

Husbands are human, too. They have feelings with which you must deal, perhaps feelings of insecurity. They may feel threatened by changes in their wives, and it takes much understanding to cope with that. But by gently, lovingly manifesting the fruits of the spirit at every opportunity, you can reassure him that his life will be better and more exciting when your weight is off. Tell him he can have a brand-new mate without going to the trouble of discarding the old one. If his response is not positive, and you can't do it with his help and for him, then you can do it in spite of him. Regardless, you *can* do it.

You have the right, the obligation, to become all that you are. And no matter what outside obstacles block your path, the largest obstacles will always lie within yourself.

There lies within self a part that wants to maintain the status quo. The flesh body, accustomed to having its own way, has no intention of giving up its gluttony without a fight. Spirit, fed by prayer and meditation, fights back. Mind, vascillating between the two, begins to feel like a referee in the Battle of Armageddon.

If Mind chooses to team up with Body against Spirit, chaos can result. Dis-ease may cause mental and physical pain that is extremely difficult to combat. Unless Spirit receives constant reinforcement, flesh will always win out—again.

This physical/mental pain is experienced most often by people who have more than 100 pounds to lose. I was one of them.

The harder I tried, the more my body resisted. My head ached. My legs felt as if the bone marrow was being drained. My back hurt. Sometimes I felt that every cell in my body was protesting to high heaven. (It was.) But through studying the Edgar Cayce readings I discovered what happens when Mind chooses to team up with Spirit through setting an Ideal.

Do first things first. . .
What is the first thing? *Self!* **and the willingness to give self; willingness to suffer in self in ideas, in the physical surroundings, for an** *ideal!***. . .[We must] dare to do the impossible.** 165-24

And further I learned. . .

. . .the true knowledge is "not of myself but the Father that worketh in me and through me." It is the knowledge that maketh alive, that maketh not afraid, that meeteth each day with the love of the greater opportunities, that maketh for the meeting of each ache, each pain within thine own body with that fortitude that makes for the removal of same through the knowledge that *He* **is God of the weak, of the great, of the lowly, of those that are in power, of those that are oppressed. And He heareth the voice of those that cry unto Him.** 262-97

Believing that it is "the Father [who] worketh in me and through me" that makes for the removal of aches and pains— even hunger pains—I continued. . .

> "Let us look within ourselves and know that we are workers together with God. We should analyze ourselves to find out just where the flesh is weak, where we are most likely to fail [and what time of day we are most likely to binge], and then seek a constant reinforcement of spirit that will make us hold on with unwavering faith to our Ideal." (*ASFG* I, p. 51)

Eventually my aches and pains subsided because *mind is the builder,* and when mind and spirit work together for an ideal the body has to cooperate.

The setting of the ideal is a Level Two activity. Getting cooperation into operation is a Level Three activity.

But here at Level One where you think you can't lose weight, you may be saying, "I can't lose weight because everything I eat makes me fat."

Cease and desist immediately; for if that is your attitude, then you are programming the body to accept that suggestion, and everything you eat will make you fat! With your next meal begin blessing food as healthful and wholesome. Bless your body and give thanks. Right away your food choices will begin to change, for it is a little difficult to feel spiritual toward eclairs and french fries. Hold a positive attitude toward food. Recognize the creative essence within. Your body cannot get along without food, so you might just as well learn to get along with it, as it is all part of the co-creative process. And recognizing ourselves as co-creators with God depends on conscious choices made through the use of the will. This leads us to a place where not only do we depend on God, but also God depends on us.

However, conscious choices made through the use of the will does not mean that you can lose weight through willpower. Willpower-induced weight losses are temporary; and that is why 90% who do lose weight gain it back. But neither can we expect God to do all the work for us. The *desire* to be thin may originate from spiritual consciousness, but once you have felt the urge to lose weight, Spirit has already moved. Now it's your turn.

Ask for guidance. You will get it. But angels don't wave wands over chubby bodies to make the fat disappear. What you *can* expect is an increased awareness of which foods to choose and which exercises to do.

Then when enough pounds have disappeared so that someone notices and asks how you did it, resist answering, "I didn't do it. God did it."

Believe me, God won't do it. He will help you to do it. But He won't do it for you. And if you think He will, you are setting yourself up for a fall. By giving God total credit for a weight LOSS, we set the stage for blaming God for a weight GAIN. Better to recognize our own cooperation with Universal Laws,

5

including the dietary ones, and see ourselves as co-creators with a loving Father, thereby accepting responsibility for our own actions. God gets blamed for everything from earthquakes to illness. Let's not blame Him for "fork in mouth" too!

Weight control depends on choices.

Choices depend on attunement with the Father.

Attunement with the Father depends on meditation.

Meditation depends on *listening*.

Move to Level Two.

Level Two

"I Want to Do It but I'm Afraid I'll Fail"
(Or succeed)

Listen to yourself as you say, "I want to lose weight but I'm afraid. . ."

Many who have a weight problem—oh, all right, *opportunity*, if you insist—talk a lot. But they don't listen. They don't hear themselves.

If we could hear ourselves discussing The Great American Pastime, "losing weight," we'd tape our mouths shut with low-calorie tape. Then we could neither speak nor eat—a decided improvement both ways.

I want to lose weight but I'm afraid. . .

. . .of my sexuality.

. . .of added responsibility.

. . .of getting sick.

. . .of having to buy a new wardrobe.

. . .of change.

. . .of life.

. . .of having nothing else to blame for my unhappiness.

One hundred pounds ago, fears such as these dominated my existence. Stress and anxiety crippled my thoughts. Occasionally it still happens.

One night, on the way from the living room to the bathroom, I stopped off at the kitchen and gained nine pounds. I tried to relieve an anxiety attack with a jar of macaroni salad. I nearly did myself in. It took me three weeks to recover from the knock-down-drag-out fight with Betty Blob, my alter ego. She emerged at Level Four. (As I was declaring *I will do it,* she was declaring, *No, you won't.)*

Listening to Betty Blob had caused me to resemble a blimp. But *hearing* her, believe it or not, has resulted in the recognition that being overweight is not the *cause* of fear, but the other way around.

Fears are dealt with more thoroughly later in this section, but for now, more background—and what a difference *listening* does make.

Thank heaven that someone listened to Edgar Cayce! And that's no mere expression. I mean *Thank heaven!* For if someone had not listened and not recorded what was said during those trance readings, not only would I not be "not fat," but I'd probably be dead.

Feeling fat was a way of life for me Before Study Group (hereafter known as BSG). My early childhood was scarred by taunts of "Fatty, Fatty, two by four, can't get through the kitchen door."

My fifth grade teacher, skinny ol' Mrs. Freeman, wouldn't let me square dance on stage because I "spoiled the looks of her group."

As a teenager, from Monday through Thursday I saved up calories so I could eat on Friday nights like a "normal" person. An early marriage and two sons by the age of 17 left me emotionally incapable of dealing with life in general, much less my constantly expanding waistline. (But on the other hand, after 25 years my marriage has proved a source of strength immeasurable. It just took a lot of growing up to recognize the value in a good one.)

After my second child was born I became so desperate that I placed myself under the care of an endocrinologist. Even now recalling the circumstances under which I found this doctor seems unreal. . .

I remember standing in front of the bathroom mirror, holding a razor blade to my wrists. The boys were playing in their bedrooms, and the thought flashed through my mind that they really shouldn't be subjected to the sight of their mother dying in a pool of blood. In my despair I must have cried out to God for help because, dazed though I was, the phone book suddenly was in my hands. As if in a dream, my finger pointed to a doctor's name in the yellow pages. I dialed the number and made an

8

appointment for the next day.

Ninety days later I was 65 pounds thinner, $750 poorer, and pregnant. But, I was alive.

Two hundred seventy days later I was 45 pounds fatter, and the 21-year-old mother of three sons.

Youth and immaturity account for much of the idiotic eating I did in those days; and, in all fairness, the doctor really did not have time to work with retraining my eating habits. The 65 pounds came off because the doctor took me off food completely and prescribed food supplement tablets, gall bladder pills, thyroid pills and diet pills. Up to 40 pills a day were rattling around in my emerging rib cage. When the pregnancy occurred, all he really had time to say as I rushed out the door to the gynecologist was, "You have to start eating again. . ."

So I did.

Potato chips, chocolate milk, mayonnaise and white bread sandwiches, sometimes with a few tomato slices thrown in for variety—all were standard fare for someone Southern born, Southern bred, and Southern fed.

By 1969 a tactless, but honest, surgeon told me I looked like a mattress with a string tied around the middle. I remember one especially masochistic day. . .sitting down, for Pete's sake—as if the measurements weren't bad enough while standing—I actually sat down and measured my hips. I even exhaled! I watched the tape register 60 inches.

What I do not remember is how I dealt with the facts of my life on that day. There I was, a 28-year-old, 240-pound mass of misery that lacked only six inches measuring horizontally what I measured vertically. To admit feeling depressed would, of course, be an understatement. But even then I must have believed that somebody somewhere had an answer for me or I would have ended it all that very day.

Somebody did.

The answers started coming in 1970 in the form of Jess Stearn's *The Sleeping Prophet,* Tom Sugrue's *There Is a River,* and Hugh Lynn Cayce's *Venture Inward.**

---

*The Sleeping Prophet, by Jess Stearn, Bantam Books, New York, N.Y., 1967.
There Is a River, by Tom Sugrue, Holt, Rinehart & Winston, New York, N.Y., 1966.
Venture Inward, by Hugh Lynn Cayce, Harper & Row, New York, N.Y., 1964.

9

By the time I waded through those three books I was hooked. I didn't care that I had been raised as an orthodox, fundamentalist, dogmatic Christian. Everything I read made sense! But it was two years later that I finally heard about an inquirer's meeting with Edgar Cayce's name attached to it.

Now keep in mind that this was BSG, so my main interests in those days were psychic phenomena, Atlantis, reincarnation, karma. . .all those neat goodies that are so much fun to study, but don't have a whole heck of a lot to do with living, *until* application enters the picture. And *application* they don't tell you about until afterwards.

So one night (it was probably a Tuesday—seems like all inquirer's sessions are held on Tuesday) I waddled into a Savings and Loan Community Room (likewise, most of these sessions are held in community rooms), and there stood itty bitty Dee Shambaugh (who might weigh 100 pounds dressed for skydiving) lecturing on the connection between the endocrine system, colors, karmic memory at cell level, energy flow, and the Lord's Prayer. I did not understand one word of any of it, but it sounded absolutely fascinating.

Dee seemed to be talking directly to me when she spoke of the spiritual centers being connected to the glands of the body, particularly the thyroid. After all, my thyroid had tested underactive all of my life—surely the reason I was fat, right? So when Dee said that meditation could balance the centers, including the thyroid, my ears perked right up.

My only experience with meditation had been sitting in a field in Ft. Lauderdale with a bunch of hippies whose main interest in life was to try to move clouds! Even then I knew better than to mess around with clouds, so I gave up. I didn't know that meditation was physical as well as mental and spiritual, and I didn't know that meditation was *listening*.

What does listening have to do with losing weight?
Everything.

For once the inner-life connection is made with the still, small voice within, the information that you need to deal with your own Betty Blob, or Sally Slob, or whatever name you will give to your alter ego, becomes accessible.

Sometimes dramatically. Such happened to me one Saturday afternoon in 1972, while I was dressing to attend a son's Little

League ball game.

Study Group had been meeting at our house for about three months, during which time we had been working with meditation. It sounded simple enough. All we had to do was sit still for fifteen minutes, quiet the body and the mind, and listen to the God within speak to us. Nothing to it.

Well, for three months I had been sitting with a mosquito biting my toe, my eyes itching, dying of thirst, hating that miserable chair and thinking every single day that I'd never get the hang of this meditation thing. But I kept at it every single day, and that's the point. Lesson number one is, "Hang in there." I did—even though I could not see one bit of good. I wasn't even sure what meditation was supposed to do except make me a better channel for God in the earth—whatever that meant. Then on that Saturday afternoon in June, I found out what that meant.

The day had passed uneventfully. Saturday chores had crowded the time, making meditation inconvenient. As I began to dress for the ball game, dreading the Florida heat—gads, it's hard to stay cool when you're fat—an inner nudge prompted me to take a couple of minutes. I figured it wouldn't hurt to be late for the game. Besides, the bedroom was air-conditioned. The ballfield wasn't. So I sat down on the floor, made my usual clumsy attempt at a half-lotus position—equally as difficult as keeping cool when you're fat—and began to try to meditate. This time something was different.

Something akin to an altered state of consciousness occurred, and a voice spoke. The exact words don't matter, but afterwards, I was certain that I would succeed at losing weight this time, where I had always failed before. It surely would be only a matter of days, weeks at the most, before I'd be ravishingly slender and gorgeous.

Needless to say I didn't exactly announce it over the loud speakers when I arrived at the ballfield. One must be very careful to whom one confesses hearing voices. But I was so certain of the authenticity, I half expected to shrink four sizes during the drive to the field. I honestly think I was disappointed when no one raved about how much weight I'd lost in the last 20 minutes.

Five years later and finally thin—well, not exactly *finally,* I've had my maintenance problems—I was and still am learning: It ain't what you *know,* it's what you *do* that counts.

Weight that could have been lost safely within a year or so took me five years to get rid of because, though I talked a good game, I had to learn that spiritual understanding without action becomes a hindrance.

Sitting around "being spiritual" and spouting platitudes doesn't work. I know. I tried it. And wound up in more trouble than ever.

This business of being spiritual can get tricky. It can hang you out on a limb and leave you feeling vulnerable, a condition that most fat people abhor, which is one reason for staying fat in the first place, as discussed in *Faces of Fear*. (See end of this chapter.)

For instance, week after week during Study Group, we talked about being of service to others. Learning to be channels of blessing, healing and help to other people would, according to the *A Search for God* books, be a way of discovering our true relationship with God. My family seemed a good place to start, only it backfired at first. For one thing *service* to my family meant, to me, cooking for them. That's all I knew; food plus food equals love. After all, nothin' says lovin' like something from the oven—just ask the Pillsbury Doughboy. Would *he* lie? And the second thing was that I was beginning to relax about being fat.

I was becoming *spiritual*, and after all, one doesn't have to be skinny if one is *spiritual*. I mean, God loves fat people, *too*, doesn't He?

Couldn't one look like a mattress with a string tied around the middle and still be beautiful on the inside, where it counts?

Another meaning of service in those days was to be calm, quiet, and peaceful (a condition completely unnatural for me), so I moved through my days "practicing the Presence" with what I'm sure must have been a glazed look in my eyes. There I was cooking and smiling and generally acting like a zombie, and being patient with the kids while they were wrecking the joint.

Then my Study Group days almost came to an end when my husband, bored to the teeth with all my spirituality, threatened to saw off that limb once and for all! Never one to mince words, he shouted, "If you don't knock off all this self-righteous junk, you can just forget about that group of *nuts* you're meeting with and let life get back to normal!"

Whoops, time to backtrack and start over. Somewhere along the line I blew it, because working with the Edgar Cayce material is, first and foremost, supposed to make one a better whatever-it-is that one is.

Then I read:

> "If self-development is our aim, then we must begin just where we are. It will do no good idly to wish to be in some other condition or surrounding; for, unless we have mastered our present one, the second state will be worse than the first." (*ASFG* I, p. 17)

That really scared me. I could not imagine a "worse state" than being a fat housewife, and now Tom was mad at me, too. There I was trying to get out of *that condition,* and things were getting all balled up. I was confused, hurt, frustrated, but I read on:

> "The first and last obstacle to overcome is understanding ourselves. Until we are fully aware of all that constitutes our existence we have no right to say that this or that is the aim and goal of life." (*ASFG* I, p. 17)

Holy cow! It could take forever to become "fully aware" of all that was constituting *my* existence—and it was *only* existence—it sure wasn't *living.*

To master the present state meant one thing: *lose weight.* And yet, something called "full awareness" had to be achieved before I could even claim the right to set goals for myself—a perplexing paradox.

But at least I was beginning to get a glimmer of why, though I'd been on every diet ever devised by mankind, I was still fat.

So I decided to shut up, sit down, and listen. Again.

And knew: The *body,* yours, mine and everyone else's, is The Temple. There *is* no other. Everything that ever was or ever will be dwells within. Jesus used a whip to clear a temple. It will be sufficient to remodel yours.

I didn't quite know how I was going to accomplish this miracle. I'd failed so many times before. But I knew one thing—I'd have to begin just where I was because wishing just was not enough. Being "spiritual" was not enough. Something was moving, and though I didn't know it yet, it was *me.*

A primary teaching of the Edgar Cayce readings is that *mind is the builder.*

We are, not *can be* or *will be*, but are what we have built with our minds, what we have *chosen*.

I was fat because I chose to be and so are you.

BSG I think that I mostly blamed my heredity, environment, and glands. What could I do? I had fat ancestors!

But Cayce won't even allow that cop-out because the information says we even chose *them!*

And while talking about listening, it's impossible not to talk about choices, because the first choice that is to be made is to sit one's fat fanny down in a chair and listen.

To what?

Well, don't expect to hear a detailed outline of what to eat in the next 24 hours. In fact, don't *expect* anything. Just sit there and repeat the Lord's Prayer silently and know that something physical is happening to your body.

The book, *Meditation and the Mind of Man,** by Herbert B. Puryear and Mark A. Thurston, could have been titled "Meditation and the Body," because meditation involves the physical as much as the mental and spiritual.

This point is best made in the third chapter of *Meditation and the Mind of Man,* entitled "Physiology of Meditation," which quotes from reading 281-13:

...there are *definite* conditions that arise from within the inner man when an individual enters into true or deep meditation. A physical condition happens, a physical activity takes place! Acting through what? Through that man has chosen to call the imaginative or the impulsive...

The question was asked of Edgar Cayce: "How should the Lord's Prayer be used in this connection?"

The answer that was given states: "As in feeling, as it were, the flow of the meanings of each portion of same throughout the body-physical. For as there is the response to the mental representations of all of these in the *mental* body, it may build

---

Meditation and the Mind of Man, by Herbert B. Puryear, Ph.D., and Mark A. Thurston, Ph.D., A.R.E. Press, Virginia Beach, Va., 1975, 1978.

into the physical body in the manner as He, thy Lord, thy Brother, so well expressed in, 'I have bread ye know not of.' " (281-29)

Review the following chart to trace the movement of the energy in the body as the words of the Lord's Prayer are spoken.

The Lord's Prayer, the Seven Centers, and the Order in Which They Open

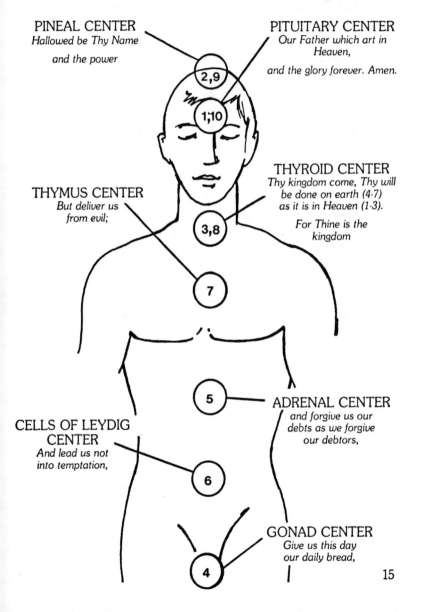

PINEAL CENTER
Hallowed be Thy Name

and the power

PITUITARY CENTER
Our Father which art in Heaven,

and the glory forever. Amen.

THYROID CENTER
Thy kingdom come, Thy will be done on earth (4-7) as it is in Heaven (1-3).

For Thine is the kingdom

THYMUS CENTER
But deliver us from evil;

ADRENAL CENTER
and forgive us our debts as we forgive our debtors,

CELLS OF LEYDIG CENTER
And lead us not into temptation,

GONAD CENTER
Give us this day our daily bread,

15

In no way am I suggesting that one should meditate to lose weight. The purpose of meditation is attunement with God. And wherever that attunement leads is holy ground.

But for me, being fat was hindering all my attempts at creativity. My feelings about being fat cost me more than one job. By mutual consent I left an interior designer with whom I was training because "my body didn't fit the image she was trying to project." She was 75 years old and chubby, herself. But she tried to surround herself with young, "with-it" looking people.

Another time I was fired because a department manager decided, after three days, that I would never catch on to the work. He didn't know that I was in pain from being stuffed into a too-small girdle and waist cincher, and that was why I couldn't concentrate. Had my feelings about being fat not prevailed, I would have just let it all hang out and dug in and done a good job.

Being fat almost cost me my marriage because I hated to socialize. Tom's advertising agency job called for hob-nobbing with the "beautiful people," one of whom I wasn't. I felt so inferior and inadequate because of being fat I just would have rather stayed home. Tom's always been blind as a bat where I'm concerned. He just didn't see the fat; or, if he noticed, he just didn't care. What he did care about, however, was having to deal with my misery which pervaded our lives. BSG I was jealous, suspicious, hateful, and just *knew* he couldn't possibly love someone like me. I was so filled with self-hate that the idea that anyone could love me was inconceivable.

Therefore, for me, attunement with God meant learning to love myself, and paradoxically, learning to be of service to Him and others *in spite of being fat*.

I couldn't get off square one until I came to grips with a couple of hard facts:

1. My whole life, including the fat, was nothing more than a manifestation of past *choices*. I was not a victim.

2. All the answers to all the questions were *within*.

Once I got those straight, through continued weekly meetings of the Study Group, it was an easy jump to the conclusion that, if through *choices* I had caused it, then through *choices* I could change it.

And if the answers were within, then the questions must be also, and the way to reach both the questions and the answers must be through meditation. However, the question to be answered was not, "How do I lose weight?" but rather, "What would Thou have me do?"

Once that question is asked sincerely, an answer is not long coming.

Be listening so you don't miss it. The answer may not come during meditation. Those fifteen minutes or so daily are but a fraction of the remaining 23 hours and 45 minutes during which we *act* on the attunement that is made. And mental awareness that an attunement has been made is not even necessary. It is enough to choose to try.

For me the answer seemed to be, "Set your house in order."

It came not so much in audible words as in becoming increasingly aware of disorder all around me. Retraining my housekeeping habits was easy. The real chaos was within me, in the form of attitudes and emotions that were much more difficult to rearrange. Unlike furniture that, when moved, stays put, attitudes, when shoved, shove back!

Impatience, for example, is an attitude that loves to push us around, especially when we are trying to do something physical, like lose weight. Medically sound weight losses of two or three pounds a week seem unacceptable at times, so impatience can push us into attempting some really stupid tricks, like starving ourselves for days on end, only to wind up stuffing afterwards, because the poor body has panicked and is convinced we are trying to commit suicide. Living one day at a time and consistently choosing the right amounts of the right foods are evolutionary processes that come with persistence, plus an understanding of ourselves as co-creators.

Listening can further this understanding because listening to the answers within can lead us to new people and situations that lead further still to others, which can lead us right back to ourselves so that we begin to get a glimpse of why we are trying to lose weight in the first place. Yes, it's a round-robin, but society's reasons just aren't good enough for making all the necessary changes involved in losing weight.

Vanity rubs our puritan consciousnesses the wrong way. I've never met a "spiritual seeker" who would go hungry for the sake of vanity. Somehow we always get hung up on "it's what's within that counts."

Health reasons don't touch us because we are convinced we can heal ourselves of anything.

We instinctively know that being slim won't make us better people or purer souls.

Most of us sense the error in the view that to be fat is a sin. Somehow we just don't buy that stuff about how the devil uses food to tempt us. The theme, "Turn Your Appetite Over to Jesus and He Will Make You Thin," just doesn't ring true for us.

I respectfully submit that Jesus doesn't give a rip if we weigh 400 pounds *if* the weight is not a hindrance to our true purpose for being here—to be co-creators with the Father.

But if we are hindered by fat, or any other condition, it is our challenge, our prime directive, to eliminate these crippling influences from our lives as much as we can.

The decision to lose weight or not is individual.

The following exercise may help you to clarify in your mind your motivations behind past choices.

Instructions

The following is an experiment in listening, but this time, instead of literally letting it go "in one ear and out the other," you will capture the inner consciousness on paper, where it can be studied and worked with constructively.

Think of this experiment as an adventure into the known—a guided journal journey. For what is more *known*, though not necessarily *applied*, than the principles of weight control?

Our society as a whole probably knows everything there is to know about losing weight. Yet our society is one of the most overweight on earth. We don't apply what we know. Eighty million of us are too fat! We blame everything from the food industry to our genes. But the Cayce material suggests that we alone are responsible for our ancestry, our bodies, even our society. So, therefore, we must conclude that we are fat because we have chosen to be. Why? Because there is a payoff for being overweight, and there is a part of ourselves that knows what that payoff is.

Here you will *ask* for insight *(and ye shall receive)* into why you have chosen to be fat.

He that hath an ear, let him hear. . .

In working with this idea of wanting to be fat, let me suggest that you write from the space between breathing in and breathing out. An inner life connection seems to be more forcefully made between these two points. Just apply the pen to the paper, and allow the words to begin to flow from this space.

Complete the following (and stop resisting—you might learn something):

I want to be fat because ⎯⎯⎯⎯⎯⎯⎯⎯⎯⎯⎯⎯⎯⎯⎯⎯

⎯⎯⎯⎯⎯⎯⎯⎯⎯⎯⎯⎯⎯⎯⎯⎯⎯⎯⎯⎯⎯⎯⎯⎯⎯⎯⎯⎯

⎯⎯⎯⎯⎯⎯⎯⎯⎯⎯⎯⎯⎯⎯⎯⎯⎯⎯⎯⎯⎯⎯⎯⎯⎯⎯⎯⎯

⎯⎯⎯⎯⎯⎯⎯⎯⎯⎯⎯⎯⎯⎯⎯⎯⎯⎯⎯⎯⎯⎯⎯⎯⎯⎯⎯⎯

⎯⎯⎯⎯⎯⎯⎯⎯⎯⎯⎯⎯⎯⎯⎯⎯⎯⎯⎯⎯⎯⎯⎯⎯⎯⎯⎯⎯

⎯⎯⎯⎯⎯⎯⎯⎯⎯⎯⎯⎯⎯⎯⎯⎯⎯⎯⎯⎯⎯⎯⎯⎯⎯⎯⎯⎯

⎯⎯⎯⎯⎯⎯⎯⎯⎯⎯⎯⎯⎯⎯⎯⎯⎯⎯⎯⎯⎯⎯⎯⎯⎯⎯⎯⎯

⎯⎯⎯⎯⎯⎯⎯⎯⎯⎯⎯⎯⎯⎯⎯⎯⎯⎯⎯⎯⎯⎯⎯⎯⎯⎯⎯⎯

⎯⎯⎯⎯⎯⎯⎯⎯⎯⎯⎯⎯⎯⎯⎯⎯⎯⎯⎯⎯⎯⎯⎯⎯⎯⎯⎯⎯

⎯⎯⎯⎯⎯⎯⎯⎯⎯⎯⎯⎯⎯⎯⎯⎯⎯⎯⎯⎯⎯⎯⎯⎯⎯⎯⎯⎯

⎯⎯⎯⎯⎯⎯⎯⎯⎯⎯⎯⎯⎯⎯⎯⎯⎯⎯⎯⎯⎯⎯⎯⎯⎯⎯⎯⎯

⎯⎯⎯⎯⎯⎯⎯⎯⎯⎯⎯⎯⎯⎯⎯⎯⎯⎯⎯⎯⎯⎯⎯⎯⎯⎯⎯⎯

⎯⎯⎯⎯⎯⎯⎯⎯⎯⎯⎯⎯⎯⎯⎯⎯⎯⎯⎯⎯⎯⎯⎯⎯⎯⎯⎯⎯

⎯⎯⎯⎯⎯⎯⎯⎯⎯⎯⎯⎯⎯⎯⎯⎯⎯⎯⎯⎯⎯⎯⎯⎯⎯⎯⎯⎯

⎯⎯⎯⎯⎯⎯⎯⎯⎯⎯⎯⎯⎯⎯⎯⎯⎯⎯⎯⎯⎯⎯⎯⎯⎯⎯⎯⎯

⎯⎯⎯⎯⎯⎯⎯⎯⎯⎯⎯⎯⎯⎯⎯⎯⎯⎯⎯⎯⎯⎯⎯⎯⎯⎯⎯⎯

⎯⎯⎯⎯⎯⎯⎯⎯⎯⎯⎯⎯⎯⎯⎯⎯⎯⎯⎯⎯⎯⎯⎯⎯⎯⎯⎯⎯

⎯⎯⎯⎯⎯⎯⎯⎯⎯⎯⎯⎯⎯⎯⎯⎯⎯⎯⎯⎯⎯⎯⎯⎯⎯⎯⎯⎯

⎯⎯⎯⎯⎯⎯⎯⎯⎯⎯⎯⎯⎯⎯⎯⎯⎯⎯⎯⎯⎯⎯⎯⎯⎯⎯⎯⎯

⎯⎯⎯⎯⎯⎯⎯⎯⎯⎯⎯⎯⎯⎯⎯⎯⎯⎯⎯⎯⎯⎯⎯⎯⎯⎯⎯⎯

⎯⎯⎯⎯⎯⎯⎯⎯⎯⎯⎯⎯⎯⎯⎯⎯⎯⎯⎯⎯⎯⎯⎯⎯⎯⎯⎯⎯

⎯⎯⎯⎯⎯⎯⎯⎯⎯⎯⎯⎯⎯⎯⎯⎯⎯⎯⎯⎯⎯⎯⎯⎯⎯⎯⎯⎯

Permit me to share some conclusions to which others have come in working with this idea:

I want to be fat because—it makes my mother unhappy.

I want to be fat because—people expect less of me.

I want to be fat because—I feel more comfortable. If I'm too thin, I stand out from the crowd, and I feel self-conscious.

I want to be fat because—eating brings more satisfaction in my life than anything else.

I want to be fat because—I fear sexual confrontations with the opposite sex. This is the most common. In fact, as you continue to work with this idea of wanting to be fat, you may uncover other fears of which you were previously unaware.

The aforementioned conclusions are all negative. But you may uncover some unconscious motivations for being fat that are positive. I know a woman who discovered that she wanted to be fat so she would feel soft to her grandchildren as her grandmother had felt to her. Baking cookies brought her great joy. So did eating cookies. Therefore, for her to try to be thin would have caused great feelings of deprivation at a soul level— feelings that stemmed from her maternal consciousness around which she has built her whole life. Her only reason for even considering trying to lose weight was societal. She felt strange because being fat did not cause her great pain. Once she got a handle on her motivations, she could face society (and her doctor) with confidence. The payoff of being fat was, to her, worth any minor disapproval she felt from others.

Her choice, instead, was to bake healthier cookies and to eat fewer of them herself. She listened to her inner self and chose. No more can be asked of anyone.

At Level Three this same type of written exercise is used to determine why we want to be thin.

But first, there are fears to face.

Deliberately choosing *not* to be thin is decidedly different from wanting to be thin but being afraid of the effort—or the results.

To many, both men and women, fat feels safer, but especially to women because men seem to feel fewer emotional complications relating to body image. Men, whether fat or thin, generally do not define their selfhood in terms of how much space their bodies occupy. From childhood women receive contradictory input concerning their roles.

On one hand a "real" woman is presented as a nurturing creature: Mother Earth, angel wings outspread, sheltering and feeding all who enter her dominion, a selfless tower of strength to whom others turn for love. Any woman who differs may be considered somewhat flawed in character.

On the other hand this same "real" woman is required to look beautiful and thin and sexy, but not too sexy. The shoulds and oughts surrounding womanhood doom many efforts to lose weight.

As a weight control columnist, I received letters—all from women—attempting to express their desires to lose weight. Running through their letters were undercurrents of fears and anxieties, often ill-defined, but unmistakable nevertheless.

Fears overlap, but the recurring themes fall into six categories, and I've added a seventh:

Fear of. . .
1. Loss of familiar boundaries
2. Appearing self-centered
3. Competitiveness and jealousy from and of others
4. Feeling too powerful or powerless
5. Imagined expectations of self and others
6. Sex
7. Perfection

Fear of Loss of Familiar Boundaries

A 45-year-old woman we'll call Jane wrote, "I need to lose about 60 pounds, and I really do do well sometimes. But lately I've noticed that whenever I lose about 25 pounds, everything begins to close in on me. . ."

This closing-in-on-me feeling occurs in women who are using fat as a protective wall against the world. The need to keep others out, to be separated from others, clashes with the need to be closer to others, producing a conflict, a paradox. By losing weight we think others can get closer to our *real* body, which we think is hiding somewhere beneath the fat. When weight loss occurs we may be left feeling vulnerable, fragile, invadable. These feelings can be terrifying.

Unless the entire body, fat and all, is first claimed as your own and acknowledged as a manifestation of past choices, any weight loss is likely to be temporary. To separate the body into two sections, one fat and one thin, is to deny self. Thinking of our true selves as being surrounded and protected by fat—rather than seeing the fat as an integral part of the whole person—blocks the ability to relate.to other people lovingly. We cannot allow anyone to get too close until we expand the consciousness to embrace all of one's self and recognize that the boundaries we place on self and others are imagined. Once we understand that boundaries are only mind images subject to our control, we no longer need fat as a barrier to keep the world from closing in.

In *A Search for God* we read:

> "We should never allow ourselves to feel separate and apart from God or our fellow man; for what affects our neighbor. . .affects us. The people of the earth are one great family. We should love without distinction, knowing that God is in all. By making ourselves perfect channels that His grace, mercy, peace, and love may flow through us, we come to realize more and more the Oneness of all creation. Let us keep the heart open that the voice of Him who has called may quicken every thought and act. His ways are not hidden nor far away, but are manifested to those who will hear and see the glory of the Oneness. Through the activity of the will is the method by which each of us should prepare himself as a channel for forces that may assist in gaining a greater concept of the Oneness of the Father in the material plane." (*ASFG* I, p. 116)

Fear of Appearing Self-Centered

Many who desire slimmer, healthier bodies have difficulty because of the time and energy expenditure involved. Always taught to put the interest of others ahead of their own, some feel conflict when attempting to merge their own need to be thin with the need to be of service to others.

Laura, a wife, mother of school-aged children, and secretary to an executive, wrote, "Every minute somebody needs something from me. I love my family and my job, but I never have time to think about myself except for being unhappy about letting myself gain 40 pounds. I hate the way I look. . ."

The implication in Laura's letter is that to give to herself the time and energy she needs to lose weight would take something away from those for whom she cares, her family and her boss. To sacrifice the needs of others for her own needs might cost her in terms of family affection and her career.

Laura's letter further indicated that she was fearful of appearing vain and selfish to others, but even more afraid of seeming so to herself. Her life was centered around service to others, and the idea of doing unto herself as she would do unto others made her anxious.

Self-involvement with thinness seemed, to her, appalling. At the same time she had needs of her own: "I love my family, *but*..."

Her need to like the way she looked created conflict. She felt she had time to love everybody but herself. Resentment can result when your own needs are always suppressed. Resentment toward those you love best *plus* anxiety about how to meet your own needs and everyone else's, too, restrict the flow of love you would naturally be able to give. Your whole life then becomes unbalanced.

Therefore, giving to your own self first, fulfilling your own desire for thinness, is liberating. Appearing acceptable to your self frees your mind to think of others, unhampered by self-recrimination. Taking care of your own needs results in being less self-centered and being more willing to go and do for others.

Repeated here from Level One is a quote from the Edgar Cayce readings:

Do first things first...
What is the first thing? *Self!* and the willingness to give self; willingness to suffer in self in ideas, in the physical surroundings, for an *ideal!*...[We must] dare to do the impossible.   165-24

Know yourself, and the truth shall set you free.

Fear of Competitiveness and Jealousy of and from Others

Negative impulses, which might be horrifying, can arise when the body starts changing. Suddenly to find yourself having to compete in a thin world, where your self-worth is ranked according to outward appearance, has sent many women screaming for sanctuary back inside a shelter of fat.

Many find being fat allows them to remain outside the arena of human emotion, where life is played out against a background of bright lights, loud music, and Pepsi Generation commercials.

Imagining themselves competing where someone is always prettier, smarter, *thinner* make some women just give up, feeling inadequate, as did Martha, who wrote, "I was an account executive for four years during which time I battled constantly to keep my weight down, so that I appeared more efficient, conscientious, and trustworthy. I got so tired of feeling judged by my appearance, I finally couldn't take it anymore, and quit.

"The first thing I did after quitting was gain 28 pounds. Now I'm contemplating trying to lose it, but I can't bear the thought of having to compete again. . ."

To Martha, and others, competition equals being thin. Maybe this is because in our society beauty and personality are saleable qualities. Beauty contestants vie for money, prizes, and glory. Cute baby contests and Queen-of-the-Prom consciousness perpetuates the myth that, somehow, beautiful is better; and somehow manages to ignore the fact that beauty is both subjective and debatable.

Also in the thin world, one may be asked to deal with jealousy from others and of others, both painful experiences. Without a sense of balance, a sense of permanence, and an understanding of ourselves in relation to others, withdrawal from society seems preferable. But in *A Search for God* we read:

> "We should let neither flattery, criticism, nor opinions of others turn us aside from those vital things for which we stand—those things that are lifting us upward and building within us that which will endure until the end. Let us turn within to see if we are being true to ourselves when temptations arise. We know that we cannot be true to others unless we are first true to ourselves." (*ASFG* I, p. 33)

Fear of Feeling Too Powerful or Powerless

One person may fear that a major accomplishment such as losing a lot of weight would give a feeling of having too much power over self and others.

Another person may fear exactly the opposite: that reducing body mass means losing the ability to overpower an imagined enemy. A feeling of frailness interpreted as weakness may accompany weight loss.

Both fears may exist in the same person.

Susan, after losing 33 pounds, wrote, "I get so happy when I realize I'm no longer fat, I feel like I could do anything! Sometimes I feel like I could fly! And it scares me, and makes me want to eat.

"Then some days I feel so tiny that I could be stepped on, like a bug. And I think I'd better eat (and get bigger) so they can see me..."

Susan's fears illustrate the point that either fear places the self-image in jeopardy. These anxieties must be balanced from within, else no significant weight loss will be permanent.

Power is not to be feared. In *A Search for God* we read:

> "The more we open our hearts as a channel of blessings to others, the more power we possess." (*ASFG* I, p. 59)

> "Knowledge is power, yet power may become an influence that brings evil, when it is not used constructively. . .Secular knowledge is man-made. The knowledge of God does not bind us to dogmas, or man-made beliefs; rather it sets us free." (*ASFG* II, p. 82)

Fear of Imagined Expectations of Self and Others

While imagined expectations from others create tension, we fear most what might be expected of us from ourselves if we were not fat.

Somehow we feel that to be thin is to be different; that we will no longer know who we are, how we'll look, how we'll react, how we'll feel. Strangeness can feel threatening to one who has trod the same path time and again. The unknown path to permanent thinness is paved with questions that begin, "What will I do if. . .?"

There is safety in sameness.

Change may necessitate additional action on our parts to live up to our personal expectations. If we believe that being fat is the only thing preventing us from achieving something else, when the fat is gone, so is our excuse.

"If I weren't fat I could be. . .

"promoted."

"elected to office."

"_____"(Fill in the blank.)

Too, we may fear that being thin would somehow prompt outside pressure to accept additional responsibilities. So we use weight as an excuse for avoiding a variety of activities that we prefer not to do.

For some it's easier to believe:

I can't get a job because I'm too fat.

I can't entertain my husband's boss because I don't have the energy to clean the house and cook a nice dinner.

I can't go to the office party with my husband because I'm too fat to wear a pretty dress.

I can't do volunteer work at the hospital because I'm so fat my legs hurt when I stand on my feet.

I can't take a Scout Troop because they don't make uniforms large enough to fit me.

There would be no sin in simply admitting that we don't want a job, hate housework, feel insecure or inadequate or uncomfortable or bored. Guilt about avoiding social and charitable functions creates even more anxiety which, in turn, compels more eating to relieve the guilt.

God does not expect of us what we do not expect of ourselves; but what we expect of ourselves, God expects of us.

In *A Search for God* we read:

> "If we would have [expect] life we must give life. If we would have [expect] joy we must make joy in the lives of others. If we would have [expect] peace and harmony we must create peace in self and in our relationships with others. This is the law, for like begets like. We do not gather olives from thistles, or apples from bramble bushes, neither do we find love in hate." (*ASFG* II, p. 38)

Neither do we plant corn to grow tomatoes.
Nor cookies to grow skinny.

Fear of Sex

Of the many fears that motivate obesity, the easiest to recognize but the most difficult to deal with is fear of the sexual nature.

Among the most poignant letters I have ever received was one from a 28-year-old woman named Jesse, who had reduced her weight by 80 pounds, but who still had 50 pounds to lose:

"I think I thought that getting fat would protect me from men. I've learned through psychiatry that I need to be protected from myself.

"My father 'touched' me when I was young. He wasn't as bad as other fathers I read about these days, but I now know he made me feel like I must be bad because even though I was only nine, I knew what he was doing was wrong. I blamed myself because, after all, he was my daddy, and he couldn't be wrong, so I must be doing something to make him act like that.

"Then when I became a teenager, boys were so attracted to me it scared me. I couldn't understand why they behaved toward me as they did because I never felt like I measured up to the other girls. My mother said boys don't act like that toward 'nice girls.' So I believed I was not a nice girl.

"After I got married, men continued to ask for my phone number. I've learned through years of therapy that it was my subconscious desire to be a moral person that made me unconsciously choose to gain weight to cover my sensuality. I neither wanted to appear sensuous to men, nor feel so to myself.

"But even getting enormous didn't help. My marriage began to fall apart and other men, who didn't seem to care if I was fat, entered the picture for a while. I was so unhappy and lonely that I stopped even trying to resist temptation. Then I had guilt piled up on top of fat that was piled up on top of guilt that began when I was a child!

"My psychiatrist keeps telling me I might as well go ahead and lose the rest of the weight because being fat didn't keep me out of trouble anyway. He says some women are sexy no matter how fat they are, and there's no reason to be fat and guilty when skinny and guilty will do just as well—if I insist on being guilty. He has persuaded me that I chose to feel guilty because it was easier (and more feasible, considering my age) to accept blame rather than look my father in the eye and say, 'Stop, you dirty, sick old man.'

"And my doctor has convinced me that most teenage girls send out signals testing their attractiveness—sort of run it up the flagpole and see who salutes—and that's normal. Also I've worked through why, under the stressful circumstances, I broke my marriage vows. (My husband broke his, too, but the marriage survived. Thank God.)

"All I want now is to forget the past and get on with it. But every time a man looks at me twice I panic. Sometimes I can reason it out and don't react by eating. Other times I go wild and eat everything I can possibly hold. I eat till I'm sick, then go to bed and wake up feeling—as Sally Struthers once said—like a beached whale.

"I did it again last night. That's why I'm writing to you. It's cheaper than a visit to the doctor. Besides, he's heard this so many times, he's frustrated with me.

"Is this going to go on forever?"

Jesse's letter was so compelling I regretted being unable to publish it in its entirety because of the length. So I contacted her privately. Our talks revealed Jesse's belief in reincarnation, but she had never been able to relate that belief to her present problems with her weight. And, of course, when talking with her doctor, the subject of reincarnation had never come up.

I liked Jesse intensely for her intelligence, her insight into herself; and I related to her desire to be a "good girl." After determining that she was ready, I took the plunge and brought up the subject of the Edgar Cayce readings. (Only two other times did I suggest to readers a study of the readings as an aid to weight control. The truths therein, especially regarding reincarnation, usually had to be couched in other language that is generally regarded as more acceptable by society. Ann Landers rarely quotes the Talmud.) Jesse had searched years for outside help. It was time for her to turn within.

Finally I wrote privately to her:

"Dear Jesse,

"Go ahead and lose that 50 pounds. If you don't, you'll never know the joy and exhilaration of being in control of your life—and your body.

"There is precious little in this world over which we can exert control, but our behavior—as related to food and sex—is within our realm. Protection from ourselves does not come through an armor of fat, as you have learned. This only comes through the setting of the Ideal, and then taking *actions* that align with the attaining of that Ideal. When opportunities, thoughts, and wishes present themselves for consideration, they can be measured by the Ideal. If they are inharmonious with what you have determined for yourself, you can choose to say no. Yes and No, when used wisely, are wonderful words. Say Yes to beautiful, healthful, life-giving foods and thoughts. Say No to ugly, fattening, life-stealing foods and thoughts. Since we are the result of the foods we eat and the thoughts we think—both within our control—we can, with practice, free ourselves from the need to be protected. As adults, protection by anyone from anything can be considered, in the broadest sense, an unwelcome limitation.

"However, as for the behavior of your father when you were a child, since you weren't protected from him, the only thing to do now is forgive him. The rest of your life depends on your capacity for forgiveness. If you remain trapped in that pattern of being a victim, you'll never be slim, nor will you ever be free. A most effective method of achieving forgiveness is to sit quietly, call the offender to mind, recall the offense, feel the pain all over again, then release it. Do this every time you think of the person who has hurt you—ten times a day if necessary—until you can recall the offender without recalling the offense. Your father was wrong. Accept that completely and allow yourself to feel peace about it. Everyone in the whole world is not wonderful. That's okay, and it doesn't make the world a bad place to be. Who knows what makes these demented men abuse their little girls? Surely it has something to do with treatment they have received back down the line somewhere. Lord knows, the havoc they wreak perpetuates itself for generations to come unless forgiveness stops it short.

"Too, our ability to *receive* depends on our ability to *give* forgiveness. Your letter indicates that you have never completely forgiven yourself for committing adultery. This you must do. The need for forgiving ourselves is equally as urgent as forgiving others. Maybe more so. Even though you have intellectually analyzed your reasons and say that you understand them, you still panic every time a man 'looks at you twice.'

"The fact that your marriage survived indicates that you are already capable of a great deal of forgiveness. I suspect that you have learned to view your husband's transgressions with an attitude of loving indifference. But somehow your own seem worse than his. That's typical of the double standard still in operation today, regardless of how liberated women are supposed to be.

"Now you are ready to permit yourself to be all that you are, including sexy-looking. You have two things going for you: (1) the setting of the Ideal; (2) that wonderful magic word, No.

"However, while No is a handy word to have around, chances are you won't need it so much as before. The setting of the Ideal actually changes your vibratory patterns. Others seem to sense your purpose and respond accordingly. This doesn't mean that your mother was right; moths flock to the flame. But you are not a flame. You are a thinking, reasoning being, capable of making choices based on your Ideal.

"Another handy thought to keep in mind is that even though you, through weight loss, become a strikingly beautiful woman, you are only one of many. Pretty faces and bodies are a dime a dozen. Being slender is not a threat any more than being fat is protection against assault. Fat is a diversion on which to focus to keep from attacking the real problem—patterns which have been built within self over many lifetimes.

"I have come to believe there is a silent sisterhood of women who served as temple slaves in lives past. These women now struggle to free themselves of subservient patterns in this life. Many are working through the liberation movement. Others merely vent their anger toward men by getting fat. Some become lesbians. Not all lesbians, of course, were temple slaves, but that is another subject entirely.

"It doesn't require much stretch of the imagination to believe that prostitutes are former slaves who have decided to get paid for what they once were forced to do for free.

"Neither does it seem inconceivable that our prisons are filled with women who commited acts of violence rather than again be subjected to the will of another.

"The point for you to remember, Jesse, is that though you once were a victim, you aren't any longer unless you allow it. Within each of us is the Christ Pattern, a pattern that is awakened through meditation and made operational through the use of the will. Focusing on the Ideal through daily meditation removes us temporarily from the mainstream of madness that has become our society. The information available through the Edgar Cayce readings and weekly meetings with a Study Group may enable you to cap off the help that you already have received from your doctor in such a way that you will be able to be entirely comfortable as a slender, free person. In a Study Group you will practice cooperation between your mind, body, and soul. You will understand what that means when you experience it for yourself, first hand.

"Let me know how you are coming along."

Jesse and I became good friends. In fact, she joined my Study Group for a while before her husband's job transfer moved her to another state.

In her last letter she wrote: "Whenever those old tapes start playing, I tell myself that if I need to punish myself I'll do it some other way besides being fat. That's too high a price to pay for anything!"

She enclosed a picture of herself looking fabulous in a pair of size 10 slacks.

Fear of Perfection

Ah, but that life would be perfect, we dream.

(No, none of my readers wrote letters expressing fear of perfection.)

What is perfection? What is the meaning of the final statement in the chapter entitled "Destiny of the Body," in *A Search for God*, Book II: "We can take only a perfect body back to our Maker"? (*ASFG* II, p. 60)

What is the destiny of the physical body?

"Our body is the temple of the living God, of the living soul. Is it to see corruption? Is it to be lost entirely, or is it to be glorified, spiritualized? As our body is a structure in which we manifest as a portion of the whole, so our body is in the keeping of its Keeper, even within us. What will we do with it? God gave us free wills. God Himself does not know what we will destine to do with ourselves, else would He have repented that He made man? God has not

31

ordained that any soul should perish. What of the body? Have we ordained, have we so lived, have we made our temple so untenable, that we do not care to have it glorified?" (*ASFG* II, p. 54)

Again, what is perfection?

"Our Lord resurrected and quickened His body. He is our pattern. So we, as He, must overcome death, overcome that transition, overcome that which is the conscious change of being in all matters, all phases, all experiences, that we may be one with Him, as He is one with the Whole." (*ASFG* II, p. 57)

That is perfection. Therefore. . .

"If we would be like Him, then we must so live, so conduct ourselves, that our body may be one with Him, and be raised a glorified body to be known as our own!" (*ASFG* II, p. 54)

For most of us, however, resurrection of the body we presently occupy seems a little far-fetched. So while working on overcoming "the conscious change of being in all matters, all phases, all experiences. . ." which will include, no doubt, walking *on* water and *through* walls, what about right now?

For most of us even a state of perfection, simply meaning that we have nothing about which to·complain, proves challenging. We get nervous if things go too right! We take ourselves too seriously. We must learn to laugh at ourselves and enjoy our efforts *and* the results.

We humans are delightful creatures. God reveals Himself to us through our humanness. Every blunder can become a blessing, every cross a crown when we trust Him. The changes we would make in ourselves hasten through developing an objective eye and a sense of detachment about our mistakes—*and* our accomplishments.

Dr. Gina Cerminara, in *The World Within*,* writes: ". . .any deviation from harmony or proportion or health is indicative of some psychic necessity somewhere." (p. 51)

---

*The World Within, by Gina Cerminara, Ph.D., William Sloane Associates, New York City, N.Y., 1957.

Therefore, it seems a worthwhile effort to develop insight into conditions that produce a compulsion to overeat. But this must be done without getting sidetracked by ego-glorification and selfishness, else the soul seems to sense it and blocks the way to physical improvement until we can handle it.

Improving our physical conditions is worthy of our energies, and it is best done by carrying through with an attitude of objective detachment.

Again, from *The World Within:*

> ". . .all of us, men and women alike, can be prompted by the long-range view of many lifetimes, to the awareness of our own obligation to strive consciously for beauty, on all levels of being.
>
> "This must be done almost impersonally, however, and without sensual attachment; in the spirit, as Cayce puts it, of 'making a perfect sacrifice, holy, acceptable unto God.' It must be done with the same sort of terrible compulsion that an artist feels to transfer some beautiful image to canvas, or a sculptor to capture some lovely proportions in stone. For unless it is done out of such an impersonal passion for beauty itself, and out of a kind of sense of obligation to render to the universe a gift at least as beautiful as the most insignificant of nature's handiwork, the beautiful body we create will become itself a terrible snare, trap, and delusion." (pp. 80-81)

Dealing with Fears

While choosing an appropriate method of dealing with fears I came into possession of a copy of *Faces of Fear,** by Hugh Lynn Cayce. The book combines Edgar Cayce's psychic readings with Hugh Lynn Cayce's 40 years of counseling, group therapy, and seminars on understanding and coping with fear.

While I was reading *Faces of Fear,* the idea of writing anything else on the subject became preposterous.

The "Conclusion" from this book is reprinted here with

Faces of Fear: Overcoming Life's Anxieties, by Hugh Lynn Cayce, Harper & Row, San Francisco, Cal., 1980.

permission, and with my humble appreciation to Hugh Lynn for his contribution to all of us who fear, and to this effort:

"Fear, indeed, has many faces. Fear patterns become so entangled in our lives that tracing causes or identifying the nature of our anxieties may become difficult. Do not become trapped by fixing your attention on possible causes. Begin to use the negative, sometimes even strangely fascinating, feelings of fear to change your life. You can transform anxiety and fear energies to constructive thought and action. My experience with self and others suggests that persistent work with the concepts explored in this book not only brings freedom from fear, but also releases new energies that lead to a richer, fuller life.

"This book has been written for you. If you were a desperately sick person, you would not have come this far. Fear is a universal pattern arising from our rebelliousness. Our thought form, the flesh body itself, blocks our perception of the real goal of existence. Yet through it, as we move in consciousness, we can come to know our Creator and a true relationship of love with our fellow human beings. We have shut ourselves off from God; we are guilt-ridden, unable to accept God's constant love for us, so we find it difficult to love ourselves or others.

"Yet guilt is itself a sign that we are capable of growth. J.F. Bugental puts this succinctly in *The Search for Authenticity**: 'Guilt is a part of the dignity of being a man. Were there no responsibility attaching to our choices, no guilt inhering in our identity, we would be inconsiderable, as unmeaningful as the chance scrawlings of a man infant.'

"The unconscious mind is a battlefield. Conflicts between aspects of ourselves create our fears. Our desires war with our tendencies to repress them; our real worlds struggle with our imaginary worlds; we are torn between our drive to be important and our sense of insignificance; we hope for acceptance but confront rejection; sometimes we want to live; sometimes to die.

**The Search for Authenticity*, by J.F. Bugental, Holt, Rinehart & Winston, Inc., New York City, N.Y., 1965.

"Fear symptoms arise from bodily stress, psychological childhood conditioning, and the stress of daily living. Fears may arise to haunt us from other lives. And we fear annihilation or punishment in death. Finally, we all, at some time in our lives, feel a sense of failure that grows out of the sameness of existence and a threat of meaninglessness.

"The Edgar Cayce readings speak to many of these fears and provide, for many people, ways to deal with them. For example, an important spiritual law can help renew our relationship with our Creator—the oneness of all force. We can begin to sense that we are parts of a whole and that we do have a part to play as children of God and co-creators with Him.

"Moreover, through prayer and meditation, we begin to awaken the real self, the soul. Our wills are aroused, and we can control the mind, the builder. As we set ideals, we can measure our thoughts, words, and actions. We can build fear-free constructive attitudes by ceasing to feel negative thought patterns; tuning up our flesh bodies through the mind; conscientiously trying to be positive and constructive in our thinking; checking our dreams to observe what we are building with the mind; using positive suggestions on self; spending time with inspirational reading; and developing a sense of humor. We can use small groups for protection, help with self-observation, and healing. And service to others needs to be incorporated into our daily action.

"No one idea, prescription, or action resolves anxiety or specific fears. Fear, as we have seen, is entangled in our flesh bodies, our minds and emotions and our spiritual lives. We need to change our patterns of life activity. Waking up helps us understand new dimensions of ourselves. Turning loose, letting go of our negative past and beginning *now* to rebuild new patterns of physical, mental, and spiritual activities can free us from anxieties and fears that hold us chained in a consciousness of inadequacy and even self-destruction. We can transform fear by remembering Christ's admonition: 'Let not your heart be troubled, neither let it be afraid.' (John 14:27)" (pp. 139-140)

Level Three

"I Can Do It. . ."

(If I want to and can find a good enough reason)

> "An ideal does not mean a goal. Rather, it is concerned with the motive, purpose, intention—in sum, the spirit in which we do whatever we have to do."
> *Meditation and the Mind of Man*, p. 97

The Edgar Cayce readings ask, "What would ye do with thy mind and thy body if they were wholly restored to normalcy in this experience?. . .Will these be used for the magnifying of the appreciation of the love to the infinite?" (3684-1)

What would you do with a great body if you had one?

Oh, yeah?

Well, maybe that's why you don't have one!

Seriously, students of the Edgar Cayce readings are asked to set ideals to live by, which differ from goals in that goals are something to accomplish, while ideals represent the spirit in which you set out to accomplish those goals.

What's more, the source of the readings clearly states that the setting of the ideal is the most important undertaking of your life.

What does this have to do with weight control? Maybe nothing, or maybe everything. But that's what we need to find out before we go any further in "trying to lose weight."

The whole world seems to be "dieting." Aren't you bored with the whole idea? Yes, of course, you are. But. . .still. . .you don't really like being fat, either.

The answer to the dilemma may lie between the pages of *A Search for God,* Book I, Chapter One: "Cooperation."

"Cooperation in the physical is defined as acting or operating jointly with others, concurring with others in action or effort. In the spiritual it is more. It is losing sight of self and becoming a channel through which blessings may flow to others. The blessing is cooperation in action. Whether in the spiritual or physical, action is necessary to put cooperation into operation—thus those who would come together for a common cause must have united action in the pursuit and realization of a common end.

"The best in life is ours, not at the expense of others, but in harmonious cooperation." (*ASFG* I, p. 23)

It is my firm belief that if we could get *cooperation into operation* we could conquer the universe, starting with ourselves. It may be only the lack of cooperation between the physical, mental, and spiritual aspects of self that has caused our weight problems. But before we can persuade these parts of self to act jointly to correct the situation, we need to look first at why we should do this. But even before we decide *why* we will do it, let's examine *if* we should do it.

Perhaps you are like the grandmother who loved feeling soft to her grandchildren. For her to attempt to remodel her temple into a sleek new version would have meant constructing a whole new value system. Her life, now filled with joy, may be prolonged because she no longer suffers from fat-related stress.

But the choice is yours, and the following may help you to take a hard look at your life, how you feel about being fat, your relationship to food, and if you truly desire to be thinner.

Q. When you get advance warning about an upcoming special event, do you immediately "go on a diet"?
Yes _____ No _____
Why? (Check as many as apply. If "No," skip to the next question.)
_____ Because there's something special hanging in the closet that I want to fit into.

_____ Because I don't want them to see how much weight I've gained.

_____ Because I'm ashamed of what my body is saying about my inner self.

_____ Because being fat makes me self-conscious, and when I'm thinner, I can relax, have a good time, and take an interest in others.

_____ Because I want them to think I look great.

Q. Have you ever cancelled a social engagement because of how you feel about being fat?
Yes _____ No _____
Why? (Check as many as apply. If "No," skip to the next question.)

_____ Because I have nothing to wear.

_____ Because I have nothing in common with them, and all they ever talk about is dieting.

_____ Because I can't let myself be seen like this. They wouldn't understand.

Q. Think about the people in your life. Examine your relationships with (check all who apply):
Mother _____ Father _____ Spouse _____ Children _____
Siblings _____ Co-workers _____ Friends _____
Other _____

Do any of these people, with whom you must relate daily, remind you constantly that you are fat? Yes _____ No _____
If yes, how do you react? (Check all that apply.)

_____ I get mad.

_____ I agree with them.

_____ I get bored with hearing it.

_____ I eat.

_____ I stop eating for a few days.

_____ I ignore them.

_____ I pretend to ignore them.

_____ I hurt.

Q. Think about your work. Examine your relationship with your work. My work is (check all that apply):
_____ Satisfying.
_____ Frustrating.
_____ Just a way to make a living, boring.
_____ Temporary until something better comes along.
_____ Challenging, exciting, fulfilling, exhilarating.
_____ So important to me that I would do it for free.
_____ In fact, I do it for free!
_____ Other _____

Q. I could be more effective in my work if I were not fat.
Yes _____   No _____
If "Yes," how? _____

_____

_____

_____

_____

Q. Have you ever been passed over for promotion or lost a job because of your weight? Yes _____   No _____

Q. In your relationships do you ever feel (check all that apply):
Loved _____   Admired _____   Respected _____
Cherished _____   Adored _____   Needed _____
Used _____   Criticized _____   Inadequate _____
Inferior _____   Other _____

Q. Do you believe being fat has anything to do with how others treat you? Yes _____   No _____
If "Yes," how? _____

_____

_____

_____

Q. What do you want out of life that you cannot have right now, exactly as you are? _____

_____

_____

_____

_____

_____

_____

Q. Would being thinner help you get it? Yes _____ No _____

If "Yes," how? _____

_____

_____

_____

_____

_____

_____

Q. How would your life be different if you were thin?

_____

_____

_____

_____

_____

_____

_____

_____

_____

Q. Examine your relationship to food. (Check all that apply.) Food is:

_____ My main topic of conversation.

_____ All I ever think about.

_____ The bane of my existence.

_____ My best friend.

_____ My worst enemy.

_____ Something to eat when I'm hungry.

_____ Something to eat to keep from getting hungry.

_____ A gift from God, the source of life.

_____ The devil's handiwork, a method of suicide.

_____ Necessary.

_____ Fun to plan for, cook, and eat.

_____ The cause of all my troubles.

_____ Comforting.

_____ The reason I'm fat.

_____ Something to fear.

_____ Something that I cannot control.

_____ A challenging opportunity to learn to *choose*.

By now you may be wondering how these questions relate to putting "cooperation into operation." Your answers to these questions may have uncovered mixed emotions regarding your desire to be thin. To accomplish any significant change it is necessary for your physical, mental, and spiritual levels to agree that the change is best for all concerned. When these three aspects of self agree, that's cooperation in operation. When there is disagreement, that's a stalemate. Nothing moves until everything—physical, mental, and spiritual—moves together.

For example, if you "go on a diet" whenever a special event is upcoming because "being fat makes me feel self-conscious, and when I'm thinner I can relax, have a good time, and take an interest in others," that motivation reflects "losing sight of self and becoming a channel through which blessings may flow to others." Certainly this desire is of the highest nature because at this special event, you may find yourself within earshot of a soul in need, for whom you may have the exact words to fill the need. Being able to forget about yourself and just being there for him or her is cooperation in action. If being thinner also makes you more loving and responsive to others, that fulfills the soul's need to be a co-creator with the Father and is a reason to proceed.

If, on the other hand, you feel that "Food is—something to eat to keep from getting hungry," there may be something in your physical consciousness that fears hunger. And the battle between the physical and the spiritual is on. Here is where the saying "mind is the builder" enters the picture. Mind is also the mediator. The physical body can be convinced that spirit is right about this business of losing weight, even though some patience may be necessary.

But if you checked "No" in answering all the questions, if you don't diet for special occasions, if you've never cancelled a social engagement because you are fat, if no one reminds you that you need to lose weight, if your work is a joy and you're reaching your potential, if your relationships are complete, and if you are getting from (and giving to) life all that you can as you are, then you may be excused from class.

Otherwise, read on.

I presume most of you are still with me, and I further presume that at least some of you are a bit confused about cooperation between the body, the mind, and the soul.

Let's take it "line upon line; here a little, and there a little. . ." (Isaiah 28:10)

And the place to begin is with the setting of the Ideal, for "when self is lost in the Ideal, cooperation is the natural result. . ." (*ASFG* I, p. 23)

Each one of us at this moment is manifesting what has been our ideal, even if we have never identified any particular word or phrase as such. Because as humans we are subject to Universal Law—which dictates that as we sow so shall we reap—it follows that, if we find ourselves fat, our seeds have been sown in the spirit of self-indulgence and gluttony.

Our bodies are thought forms, and, as such, can be *re-formed* by different thoughts. To find a direction for these thoughts, we look within for a word or a phrase that represents the highest understanding we have of the God within.

Again we turn to *Meditation and the Mind of Man:*

"The most important thing we can do—in whatever situation we find ourselves—is to choose the word that awakens in us the spirit of the highest that we know. What is the one word that calls forth from us the spirit in which we want to live our lives, the spirit that we would like to have motivating us?

"One reason that setting the spiritual ideal is so vitally important is that everything we perceive in the material world has as its basis some spiritual ideal. All physical manifestations have their origins in mental patterning, and those mental patterns are founded upon the impulse of a spiritual ideal." (p. 99)

Therefore to lift ourselves up and away from negative impulses that are governing our bodies, we will specify an ideal of spirit.

Ideals are, of course, applicable in every area of our lives, family, job, friends, church, etc., but for our purposes here, we will examine our ideals in relationship only to our bodies and food.

The following model is one of the more effective ways for working with ideals. Perhaps you have worked with this circle method before, and you divided the circles into pie shapes representing various areas of your life with which you wanted to work.

Here you will focus on your own body, not that any real separation can or should be made between our bodies and the rest of our lives, but rather in recognition that the experience of oneness within our own body, mind, and soul may hasten the experience of oneness with the Father, the ultimate Ideal, as suggested in the Edgar Cayce readings.

BODY

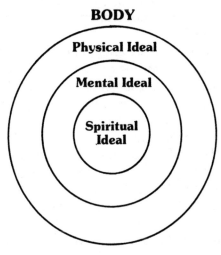

In working with these circles, keep in mind that goals do not enter in. The tendency is to think of the physical ideal as a number on a scale, or a measurement on a tape, or a dress size. Rather think of the *physical ideal as actions* you will take to reflect the spiritual ideal. The *mental ideal* has nothing to do with I.Q., but rather the *attitudes* which will direct the physical actions

The spiritual ideal is the word that defines *why* certain attitudes will be held and specific actions taken. For example, the mental response to the spiritual ideal of love might be discipline, for instance. (To express the ideal of love to my body I will think thoughts of discipline, which will direct me to eat healthful foods and do exercises.)

Before writing your word in the center circle which follows this section, hold a little dialogue between your mind and spirit. Begin with the question at the beginning of this chapter. Study this example, then try writing one of your own.

Mind: Well, what would you do with a great body if you had one?

Spirit: *I'd direct it into service for the Lord. He needs all the help He can get, you know.*

Mind: What, specifically, would you do?

Spirit: *Specifically, anything that needed to be done. He would tell me what to do if I asked. I haven't asked because without you guys' cooperation I'm pretty limited.*

Mind: Limited, how?

Spirit: *By all this internal bickering. I keep nudging you about all this extra weight we are carrying around, and you keep promising to do something about it. But every time you get serious about it, our old buddy, Body, with all those raging fat cells. . .well, you know how hard it is to get them to calm down.*

Mind: Boy, do I ever! But I think I'm ready to offer you my full cooperation. Between the two of us, old buddy, Body, won't have much choice. It'll have to come along for the ride. Maybe we can even persuade Body that it will enjoy the change.

Spirit: *Sure we can, together we can accomplish anything.*

So it might as well be something He wants us to do, do you agree?

Mind: Yes, I agree. I have about decided that creating on my own is not really satisfying. I might as well connect with the Source and really be good for something. How do we get Body to cooperate?

Spirit: *It won't be easy, but every day you sit Body down and ask it to be still. Then you repeat the Lord's Prayer over and over. With all Body's faults, the pattern of you-know-who. . .*

Mind: No, who?

Spirit: *Jesus, the Christ. . .*

Mind: Well, why didn't you just say so?

Spirit: *Never mind. The pattern is there within the cells, just waiting to be awakened. All you have to do is repeat the words of the prayer and then direct your attention to a word I'm going to give you. I'll do the rest from here. It's easier for me because I'm not as separated from Him as you are. Remember how tickled you were when I told you that placing a separation in the word Father made it read Fat Her? Anyway, I'll direct from here, you will obey, and Body will just have to go along with the program.*

Mind: Okay, but I'm confused. What is this word and how do I begin.

Spirit: *For starters, let's begin with the word SERVICE. Let's call this word our spiritual ideal.*

Mind: But I like the word FREEDOM better.

Spirit: *Yes, you would. Okay, I'll go along with that, but let's combine the two and use the phrase FREE TO SERVE.*

Mind: I like that. It has a nice ring to it. I think I can take that and run with it.

Spirit: *All right. You start holding thoughts that relate to being free to serve, thoughts like being persistent and consistent, and patiently willing to go and do. These thoughts will become our mental ideal. I'll be watching for opportunities to practice our principles, and as we get better at it, we'll find new challenges.*

Mind: Sounds good to me, but are you sure Body is going to agree with us?

Spirit: *Leave Body to Him. You just sit Body down in that chair and repeat that prayer and think about being Free to Serve. HE will take care of Body. After all, He made it originally. He knows more about how to remind Body of the Original Intention than either you or I. If we understood better, we would never have let Body get in this condition in the first place.*

Mind: Do you think Body is going to enjoy being in service to Him? And what can we feed Body to hasten the transition?

Spirit: *Yes, Body will begin to love being in service so much that before long, Body will begin nudging you about sitting in that chair. And Body will especially love the new foods it will be getting, and the exercise you will be giving it. It will take a little practice, but before too long we will be moving as one unit, in full cooperation with each other— and Him. But to answer your question as to what to feed Body, I'll be guiding you every day, so you just be listening.*

Mind: It's a deal. When do we get started?

Spirit: *We just did.*

Get a pencil and separate sheet of paper and try writing your own conversation with your spiritual self. As with all inspirational writing, try to write from the space between breathing in and breathing out.

This exercise can be very helpful in identifying a word that represents the ideal.

When completing the dialogue between mind and spirit, you are ready to complete the circle. Working from the standpoint of an ideal, rather than a mere idea, leads to internal revelations that produce external transformations.

Actually writing down the ideal helps to firm up the commitment to spiritual development and physical transformation.

The following model might be helpful in completing the circle as it relates to Body.

Example

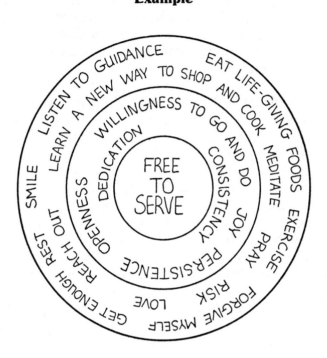

While working with the circle, keep in mind these words from *Meditation and the Mind of Man:*

"The Edgar Cayce readings stress that to set an ideal and then to make no effort to become one with it only accentuates an awareness of separation. The Christ pattern is one of integration, not division. Setting a direction for growth without making some movement in that direction serves only to increase a sense of fragmentation within ourselves. Jesus expressed this principle in His teaching, 'No man, having put his hand to the plow, and looking back, is fit for the kingdom of God.' (Luke 9:62) If we set our sights upon a new orientation and the work it will entail, and then look back to the old ways and fail to do the work of application at hand, we make it much more difficult to grow into a higher state of consciousness.

"In a sense, a statement of direction does not become an ideal without serious self-involvement. Such involvement is attained only by direct experience. In the experiencing and the application of the motivational spirit we wish to express, it becomes not just a theory of the mind, but an ideal." (p. 103)

It is doubtful that Dr. Puryear and Dr. Thurston were thinking of application of spiritual principles to weight control when writing those words, but in no area of one's life are they more applicable. *Setting a direction for growth* or, in this case, determining that there is a spiritual basis for remodeling this body temple, then not taking action in that direction, increases *a sense of fragmentation within ourselves* as little else can.

The need for *serious self-involvement* was expressed differently by Violet Shelley, author of *Reincarnation Unnecessary,* when at a lecture one day she offhandedly mentioned a "credibility gap between the conscious and the unconscious minds."

"We say that we want to lose weight, then turn around and eat a candy bar. The unconscious hears our words, but knows by our actions that we don't mean what we say, therefore, it refuses to help," she said.

In order to close this credibility gap, it is necessary that we *act,* that we "lose sight of self and become a channel of blessings to others. And that blessing is cooperation in action."

Before going on, stop here to complete the ideals circle. . .

The following is an exercise in writing a clear statement of intention about our bodies.

Once again think of this experiment as an adventure into the known. For we are calling upon an aspect of self that knows us better than we know ourselves and stands ready to aid in any endeavor that is in line with the ideal which we have set for ourselves.

Simply fill in the blanks and complete the following statement.

My body is the temple of God, and the ideal on which I will act is

My soul's need is to fulfill its role as a co-creator with the Father. For this to happen, my soul requires full cooperation from mind and body; therefore, I will eliminate all conditions which hinder the soul's purpose, including, if necessary, all excesses, especially excess weight.

I want to be slim because _____

_____

_____

_____

_____

_____

_____

_____

_____

_____

_____

_____

_____

_____

_____

_____

_____

_____

_____

_____

_____

_____

_____

_____

Level Four

"I Will Do It. . ."
(If I can just figure out *how.*
Isn't there some secret?)

You were just given the secret to being slim. Did you miss it?

When the Ideal is set, you know *why*. Motivation is a four-syllable word for *why bother*. The Ideal that you have set for yourself is why to bother. When you know why, all that's left is *how*.

Simply stated, put the Ideal first in your life.

Eventually balance between the body, mind and soul forces will result; but not unless and until you temporarily commit your whole being to acting on what you know.

That means recognizing every excuse to overeat as a cop-out, a subconscious con, the body trying to maintain the status quo by resisting changes in cellular consciousness. It further means rearranging priorities, reconditioning thinking, re-establishing the relationship to food.

Wouldn't it be nice never to read another diet book, go on another diet, dread another social occasion or lecture from your doctor or dressing room mirror?

Sounds wonderful, yes?

Sounds simple?

Hardly.

Changing priorities, attitudes, emotions, and relationships is never easy. Though the market is glutted with diet books that promise to reveal The Secret, *something is missing*. Seventy billion dollars each year are spent by people trying to learn what to eat and not eat. Fat is big business. Besides book sales, there are diet clubs, diet doctors, and every corner drugstore offers sure-cure fat fighters.

I paid a fortune to doctors, trying to find the missing element. I swallowed every pill, bought every product, and joined every flab-fighter fellowship I ever heard about. Nothing worked.

Once after polishing off a whole box of that reducing candy in a day, I threw myself through the door of a Weight Watchers meeting. I had already abandoned TOPS and Overeaters Anonymous. But even Weight Watchers, so helpful to so many, couldn't help me. Something was still missing. And I was still fat. So when one has looked everywhere and tried everything, where does one turn?

Within.

. . .ye are part and parcel of a universal consciousness or God...   **2794-3**

For thou art indeed a god in its making. . .   **1440-1**

It seemed to me that a "god in the making" ought to be able to find out how to lose weight! But there is a secret. And it is twofold:

1. Discover *why* (through the setting of the Ideal).
2. *Act* on what you already know.

The information you now have about nutrition and exercise must be *applied*. Begin with such common advice as to stop eating sugar and refined carbohydrates. Walk more. Do what you know to do. And if you hear yourself say, "I really shouldn't eat this," then *don't*.

> "We must show by our actions in our daily lives that we
> believe, that we have faith, and that we know as we use
> what we have, more will be given." (*ASFG* I, p. 49)

Show whom?
Ourselves.
More will be given by whom?
By whatever name you call God, the inner guidance that is the natural result of daily meditation. As we pray for the will to do God's will, help comes from everywhere.

"Within each of us there are certainly great storehouses of abilities and capacities which we have never used." (*ASFG* I, p. 31)

The ability to choose foods wisely can be developed with practice.

The tendency is to wait until we feel like doing something before doing it. But psychology experts agree that the greatest accomplishments are achieved by people who develop the capacity for *doing* regardless of lackadaisical feelings.

Edmund Burke said: "Never despair, but if you do, work on in despair."

A Search for God states:

"Be what you seem. . .Be what you pray to be made." (*ASFG* I, p. 34)

"Let us determine within ourselves that a constructive program will be followed [at least for today]. The conditions of this program, then, require that a definite stand be taken by each of us. We are determined that we will adhere to it, no matter what we may suffer mentally or physically. We will trust in the divine Force within for the strength to endure and for the ability to say no when we should." (*ASFG* I, p. 37)

The same Force that prompts the desire to accomplish anything can be trusted, at least until our own selfishness takes over, to lead us where we want to go.

"For us to be aware of our physical desires and appetites is physical awakening. To satisfy them selfishly is sin." (*ASFG* I, p. 36)

If our Ideal directs us into service to God, then is it not selfish to permit any condition that detracts from our ability to serve? God works through us if we so desire, whether fat or thin. But why not give Him all the energy possible with which to work?

"When we become aware that the mind can control the physical desires, then we have a mental awakening." (*ASFG* I, p. 36)

Our unwillingness to eat destructive foods may increase along with our awareness of the Ideal.

> "When we are conscious that we can reconcile the spirit within with the spirit without and know that they are one and are from the same source, God, then we have a spiritual awakening." (*ASFG* I, p. 36)

Now we may begin to make the right food choices without having to think about it.

> "As we cultivate the ability to discriminate between right and wrong, good and evil, we are reaching the plane where we may be masters of our destiny." (*ASFG* I, p. 33)

And masters of our stomachs.

> "Let us turn within to see if we are being true to ourselves when temptations arise." (*ASFG* I, p. 33)

Then look in the mirror. Temptations sometimes lose their charm when we are being true to ourselves and are seeing ourselves as we actually are, which some of us will go to any length *not* to do!

As the number one champion self-deluder of all times, I honestly did not know how I looked to others when I was fat. I made that statement to an audience one night, and a lady with an incredulous look on her face asked, "How could you not know?"

"Madam," I said, "had I known, I surely would have leaped from the nearest bridge."

I managed to hide my capacity for self-deception from myself until after I had lost weight.

Like almost all new skinnies, buying clothes was fortunately a temporary obsession. However, as I was trying on a new dress at home one day, I caught myself stooping to see how it looked in the full-length mirror. Suddenly it hit me that I could not see my head in the mirror, only my body. A quick check of every other mirror in the house revealed that in not one of them could I see my whole self! When hanging the mirrors, I had positioned each one either low enough so that only my body showed, or high enough so that I could see only my head. Good Lord, I had decapitated myself! I had conveniently disconnected my head from my body, thereby disclaiming the image.

Most of us at one time or another hold whatever self-image is necessary for self-preservation. But the Edgar Cayce readings encourage honesty in our dealings with ourselves.

> "Let us dare to see ourselves as others see us. It is well
> to stand aside and see ourselves go by." (ASFG I, p. 34)

Honesty can be painful. Many a diet has begun immediately following a photo session.

But even those who are the most determined to stick it out—no matter what—can get sidetracked when something urgent occurs unexpectedly.

A couple of times when I was losing, I found myself pacing a hospital corridor at midnight, praying for an injured child—a genuine emergency. At times like these the last thing on our minds should be food. But unfortunately these are the very times when old habits may return.

Gerri Watts, Director of the Florida Diet Workshop, says she never really had confidence that her 90-pound weight loss was permanent until she suffered three major tragedies within three months—and only regained two pounds.

"Until then," she said, "I always subconsciously feared regaining the weight. But after living through those three months and realizing that I had been automatically choosing the correct foods through it all, I knew—finally—that I would never be fat again."

Automatic, unconscious responses that align with the Ideal are developed with practice, as is faith:

> ". . .hold fast to that which we have purposed in our
> inner selves, knowing that no emergency in a material
> way or manner may arise that cannot find its solution in
> spiritual inspiration, for His promises are sure. (ASFG I,
> p. 43)

Yet for some people most of the time and possibly even most people some of the time, a smorgasbord can be an emergency. That's when:

"Keeping the channel clear, open, and ready to be used, we see the seemingly impossible begin to take place [the zippers zip] and we come to realize that no weapon that is formed against us shall prosper." (*ASFG* I, p. 59)

Not even hospital candy machines at midnight!

The deadliest weapons against us are formed, of course, within our own selves. Sometimes we use these weapons against ourselves to block the path to the unknown because we are afraid of what we might find, as we discussed in the section on fears. At other times these weapons manifest as thought forms, which we carry with us and must recognize as parts of self if we are to ever move from the "I Will" consciousness into the "I Am" consciousness at Level Five.

These thought forms can become so real that they are like another person living inside us, an alter ego.

Ladies and Gentlemen, I'd like to introduce my alter ego. Her name is Betty Blob, and she lives in a cage in my head.

You remember her. She's the one who made me eat the macaroni salad back at Level Two.

Betty Blob is to me what the devil is to Flip Wilson. She always makes me do it.

When I.shared her with the readers of my newspaper weight control column, I received a half-dozen phone calls and letters from women who admitted that they, too, had an alter ego. One reader wrote:

"I feel like you looked into my head and wrote that column about me. I think I'll name my thought form Sally Slob."

Not too long after Betty Blob emerged in my consciousness, I attended a lecture by Hugh Lynn Cayce. I remember chuckling to myself as I heard him say: "Never feed a thought form. The only way to get rid of these monstrosities is to starve them to death. Otherwise they'll just get bigger and bigger and take over your life. These things feed on our thoughts. They take our thoughts and turn them into ammunition to be used against us!"

Hugh Lynn didn't know it, but he was talking to me. After that I tried to ignore Betty Blob. But she would rattle the cage door, screeching, "Let me out of here! You can't do this to me, you skinny twerp. I'm starving to death, and I've got to eat!"

For a while, I would double-bolt the cage door so that she

couldn't escape. Then she got sneakier—and skinnier—and she learned to slip quietly through the bars. She gets skinny when I get skinny, and she *hates* being skinny. She would take hold before I was aware of her presence, and it would be 12 pounds later before I even knew she was loose.

When ignoring her didn't work, I tried hating her. But that didn't last long because there's something rather pitiful about her. Touching. . .almost. I tried to think of her as evil, but she's not really, just confused.

No amount of talking helps because she won't listen. I've reasoned, cajoled, pleaded with her to see my side. She responds with ridicule: "After all, you're no 18-year-old. What difference does a few pounds make?"

"But Betty Blob" (I always call her Betty Blob—never just Betty), "those few pounds will soon be many pounds, and that makes the difference between really living and only existing!"

But she insists that eating is more fun than anything else.

I've tried everything short of exorcism to evict her. She's no dummy, and she is good at getting what she wants. And what she wants is to be fat.

Betty Blob loves *being* fat.

But Linda Lean loves being *not fat*.

So one day I was pondering deeply why in the world I could not rid myself of this part of myself that has wreaked utter havoc in my life. Happily, I discovered that she has been truly useful to me in several ways.

Possibly she has shown me how to be a little more compassionate. It isn't difficult to equate weight control problems with alcoholism, drug addiction, and physical handicaps. Each offers opportunities for learning to love.

Furthermore, I'm not sure that without her, I would have made half the effort to learn patience with myself and others. She has shown me things about myself that my best friend—or my worst enemy—wouldn't dare.

Therefore, whenever I'm aware that we are still together, she and I, though it isn't easy, I just try to say, "Okay, Linda. You didn't get it right yet. There's something more to learn here or else you wouldn't be bulging at the seams again."

Anyway, she keeps me humble.

Valerie Harper, of "Rhoda" fame, made a point about gaining

and losing the same ten or twenty pounds repeatedly, in an interview published in *Parade* magazine:

"I get such a thrill out of losing weight that when I get so skinny there's nothing left to lose, I feel like there's nothing to do. So I gain some of it back just for the thrill of losing it again. I just love that feeling of accomplishment," she said.

Such an honest observation signals the attainment of great personal insight that, according to the Edgar Cayce readings, heralds the breaking away of barriers that stand in the way of our development.

"To know ourselves is not only to be cognizant of the acts of our physical bodies [such as what the hand sticks in the mouth], but to know ourselves as entities, complete factors, capable of knowing all that goes on within and without. [If it goes within, it shows without.] This spring of knowledge is tapped only by those who are willing to pay the price. [Even to face the truth, the whole truth.] The price is a complete surrender of ourselves, with a purification and a dedication that come only through prayer, meditation, and service [meaning *action*]. It is along the straight and narrow way, but it is open to all. The water of life is offered freely. [That's *water*, not milkshakes.] (*ASFG* I, p. 31)

It's a short hop from the "I will" consciousness to the "I am." Turn the page and get going.

Level Five

"I Am Doing It. . ."
(And learning more about myself than I wanted to know. . .)

I wish I could say that This Is the Only Way to Lose Weight. But you and I know that would be too simple. No. In weight control, as in life, it's those blasted *choices* that make it tough.

Therefore, the following is not carved in stone.

But keep in mind that everyone who has ever lost weight and kept it off has gone through these processes in one form or another.

Successful slimmers publicly make such statements as, "Oh, I found this great new diet"; "Oh, I just stopped eating"; "Oh, I joined the spa." But rarely do they offer reasons *why* they lost weight.

Nobody ever says I lost weight so that I could be of greater service to God.

When was the last time you heard a newly slender person admit that they lost weight to short-circuit a growing suicidal tendency? Life is tough enough without hanging one's pain out on a limb for public viewing. But for nearly everyone the battle has been long, hard and intensely personal, the mental processes involved complicated. That's why capturing your feelings on paper is so important. Some people claim they don't have to know where they are to get where they are going, but for most of us it sure helps.

Chances are you've lost weight before, but regained it. You

may lose weight again on a preplanned diet, or you may design your own diet. Any diet or eating plan that is nutritionally sound will work and keep you healthy, *as long as you stay on it.*

Who breathes, who is fat, who never had *any* success in losing weight on *some* program? Is there a fat person in existence who hasn't at one time or another joined Weight Watchers, TOPS, Overeaters Anonymous, or *some* program? Whose bookshelves do not runneth over with weighty tomes from Atkins, Pritikin, Simmons, and a host of other ex-fatties?

The question is: If you tried it and it was working for you, why didn't you stick with it?

The answer may be found back at Level Two where you didn't want to succeed or were afraid to succeed. Or the answer may be that the Thou Shalt Nots didn't make sense. Or perhaps the program seemed temporary, despite claims that This Is a Way of Life. With some of the programs I tried, the idea of living and eating like that forever was overwhelming, and I quit without giving it a fair chance.

Complete the following to recall to memory a time when success was on the horizon (and why it never came any closer).

I lost weight before when I _____

_____

_____

I stopped losing and/or gained it back when I _____

_____

_____

Okay. Something was working for you once before. Why did you stop?

I stopped because _____

_____

_____

If you are being honest, and you now have it straight in your mind why you stopped doing something that was working for you, consider returning to whatever that was, plus using this book to supplement that program or activity.

In the meantime, consider the following.

How to Choose a Gauge of Progress

Progress can be measured by weight, measurements, clothing sizes, feelings, and appearance. Choose a gauge to measure your progress regularly.

To Weigh or Not to Weigh

Whether or not to use the scale as a progress gauge is a personal choice. Here are four approaches to consider:

1. Don't. The weight won't weigh away, so why bother.

2. Weigh every morning. Daily weight checks are excellent aids to self-knowledge. Understanding body fluctuations is important because it eliminates panic due to normal cyclical changes. Some experts state that a refusal to face the scale indicates the onset of terminal self-delusion.

3. Weigh once weekly. The scale as a monitor is helpful if one has access to the same scale at the same time of day each week. Opponents view weekly weighing as dangerous because of the inevitable depression should one not see a change after a whole week.

4. Jump on the scale three times a day. Used mainly by persons who have shed many pounds, this approach is threefold:

    (a) The morning weight sets the tone for the day and dictates what shall be eaten that day.

    (b) The afternoon weight serves as a reminder of a commonly held belief, "that you're either getting fat or getting thin at all times."

    (c) The late-night weight reinforces the mood set by the afternoon weight and determines whether one is permitted to sleep that night. (Many midnight joggers are three-times-a-day types.)

Clothing Sizes

Some choose to gauge progress by what size clothes they are able to fit into. This is acceptable as long as the articles of clothing don't stretch. Almost everyone wears a wide range of sizes depending on the style and manufacturer. However, zeroing in on one special dress or pair of pants and making that item a goal can be be equally effective as watching the numbers on the scale.

Measurements

If measurements become the gauge of progress, make sure of three specifics:

1. That the tape measure is the non-stretchy type.
2. That you don't cheat by pulling the tape a little tighter than the previous week.
3. That you measure enough areas of the body to register some progress somewhere each week. (See the "Reality Chart" following.)

Feelings and Appearance

Less specific, but equally tangible as numbers on a scale or tape measure, are distressing emotions and attitudes toward yourself because of excess weight. Disgust, hatred, loathing are familiar companions to those who are overweight, and also to those who see themselves as overweight, but who are really not.

If negative emotions pervade your daily life, choose elimination of these emotions as a goal. (Working with the self-image building journal will help.)

If you feel okay about yourself until you look in the mirror, choose improvement in your appearance as a goal. Happily, this goal can begin to be achieved instantly through different clothing styles and better posture, regardless of how much weight you have to lose. The first impression that we make on others either enhances or blocks our ability to relate constructively. An immediate improvement in the image we project occurs when we stand erect and smile. Positive feedback from others then makes it easier to proceed to reach other more measurable goals.

Goals

On the following chart, record which gauge you have chosen to measure your progress. Fill in the applicable area of the chart, recording both *what is* and *what will be*.

REALITY CHART

Weight _____Goal _____

Measurements:

Bust _____Goal _____

Ribs _____Goal _____

Waist _____Goal _____

Navel _____Goal _____

Hips _____Goal _____

Fanny _____Goal _____

Left Thigh _____Goal _____

Right Thigh _____Goal _____

Clothing Sizes:

Blouses _____Goal _____

Pants _____Goal _____

Dresses _____Goal _____

Feelings:

Now I feel _____

_____

I would rather feel _____

_____

Appearance:

Realistically, the impression I project is _____

_____

Realistically, I would choose to project _____

_____

_____

62

Pitfalls to Pinpoint

On the following chart identify as many pitfalls as you currently recognize. Focusing on these troublesome areas may be sufficient to expand your awareness enough to offer solutions. Update the chart as necessary.

Review these pitfalls from time to time as you proceed. Solutions to each of these problems have been found by every person who has experienced permanent weight loss.

My binge foods are:

Starches, specifically _____

Salty foods, specifically _____

Sugars, specifically _____

Other, specifically _____

My time of day when I absolutely have to eat is:

Morning, specifically _____

Afternoon, specifically _____

Evening, specifically _____

Late night, specifically _____

My tendency to overeat increases when:

At work, specifically _____

At social occasions, specifically _____

At family occasions, specifically _____

At home alone, specifically _____

With certain persons, specifically _____

With certain situations, specifically _____

Other, specifically _____

_____

63

My recognizable fears center around (check all that apply):

Loss of familiar boundaries _____

Appearing self-centered _____

Competitiveness and jealousy _____

Power (too much or too little) _____ (vulnerability)

Expectations of self and others _____ (responsibility)

Sex _____

Perfection _____

Relationships with:

      Men _____

      Women _____

      Parents _____

      Children _____

      Friends _____

      Others _____

      All of the above _____

Calories and/or Carbohydrates: To Count or Not to Count

As in choosing a gauge of progress, again you choose a method of weight control. There are different approaches to counting calories and carbohydrates to be considered:

Some see counting calories and/or carbohydrates (and in some cases, proteins) as too tedious, boring, and time-consuming to be of real value to the permanent life changes that accompany permanent weight control.

Others feel that counting, especially counting calories, provides peace of mind as nothing else, and that going to sleep knowing you didn't blow it is worth the trouble.

Which Diet?

"Diet," in some circles, has become a four-letter word. However, Webster's definition for diet is simply: "what one *normally* eats or drinks."

This removes the temporary, fad, or shortlived connotation that the word diet currently carries.

One's diet, therefore, can be molded, altered, and changed according to personal preferences and tastes (and by which fresh foods are in season). And certainly it never needs to be boring, dull, or rigid.

Every week there's a new "diet" published for the purpose of selling magazines and books. Most of these are destined for the scrap heap even before the ink is dry, and justifiably so. That does not mean some of these fads don't produce weight loss. Some do. I ought to know. I tried them all.

Diet-hopping used to be my favorite game. And if I managed to get from one diet to another without regaining all I'd lost in between, so much the better. But the anxiety of "will it work or won't it?" drove me nuts. I always had the feeling that this, too, is temporary, and worrying about it became unbearable. So finally I designed my own diet, which I will share with you later.

The question, then, of which diet is not easily answered. What is right for one person is not necessarily right for another. Yet many food programs have merit.

The consciousness of the individual makes one diet more effective than another. But all good is from God. All food is from God. If you doubt that a food is indeed *not* from God but rather from a chemist's lab, then don't eat it.

The only method of choice concerning foods is through one's own consciousness.

That thou eatest, see it doing that thou would have it do. Now there is often considered as to why do those of either the vegetable, mineral, or combination compounds, have different effects under different conditions. It is the consciousness of the individual body! Give one a dose of clear water, with the impression that it will act as salts—how often will it act in that manner? 341-31

In a weight-control class I was conducting was a woman whose consciousness directed her to wash all her food in a mild Clorox solution to cleanse away the poisons. She also spoke freely of an intense hatred between her and her husband, and said she did not expect to lose weight until after his death. This woman believed in reincarnation, and she freely elaborated on the details of the "negative karma" between her and her husband. Also she remembered having starved to death in a previous life; therefore, she could not tolerate hunger in this life.

Another woman in this same class shared her feelings about having been rationed food during the Depression. "I will not be told what I may and may not eat—ever again!" she said. "I must permit myself to eat what I want, but allow myself to *stop eating,* also, knowing that there is plenty of food available to me if I want it."

Both these women have experienced true hunger. The first in a previous life, the second in this life. The first woman admitted that she has never known hunger in this life: "Once I tried to fast for 24 hours, and after 8 hours without food I panicked and would have become hysterical had I not broken the fast," she said.

Neither woman could ever tolerate hunger, obviously, but both women desired to be slim. The advice to them both was the same: to make vegetables the main staple of their diets. Vegetables and fruits will not prohibit weight loss!

While physical hunger is real, psychological hunger is equally demanding. Sometimes just nothing will satisfy unless it is salty, warm and creamy, cold and sweet, sour, or tangy. But even these specific demands can be met without undoing all efforts to lose weight.

If your mouth is saying, "It's gotta be salty!" and you're trying to lose weight, which food do you choose: dry roasted peanuts at 600 calories or more per cup, or a 15-calorie pickle?

If mouth is craving warm and creamy, which do you choose: 400-calorie potato soup with butter and thickener, or 100-calorie potato soup made with dry skim milk and butter salt?

Mouth says cold and sweet. What will it be? A big juicy, luscious ripe pear, an apple, artifically sweetened ice tea, or ice cream. Which choice does your consciousness permit?

Designing Your Own Diet

Then the diet: This should be not so rigid as to appear that you can't do this or you can't do that, but rather let the attitudes be— everything that is eaten, as well as every activity—purposeful in conception, constructive in nature. Analyze that! Purposeful in activity, constructive in nature! **1183-2**

What has come to be known as the "Cayce Principles of Food Combining" turns out to be the perfect balance for weight control!

Eighty percent of the diet should be alkaline-producing foods. Twenty percent should be acid-producing foods.

Review the list below with an eye for the low-calorie foods.

ALKALINE-PRODUCING FOODS (80% of the diet)

Eggs (yolks only)

Fruits (all fresh and dried except cranberries, plums, and large prunes)

Milk (all forms)

Vegetables (all fresh and dehydrated, except legumes and rhubarb)

ACID-PRODUCING FOODS (20% of the diet)

Animal fats	Kidneys
Beef	Lamb
Brains	Lentils
Bread	Liver
Chicken	Peanuts
Coconut	Pecans
Corn meal	Pork
Dried beans	Rhubarb
Dried peas	Sweetbreads
Duck	Syrup
Egg (whites only)	Turkey
Filberts	Vegetable oils
Goose	Walnuts
Grains	White sugar
Hearts	Wild game

Following is the Diet Review Sheet, courtesy of the A.R.E. Clinic, Inc., Phoenix, Arizona. This summary of the principles of the Edgar Cayce readings is recommended for maintenance-level weight control.

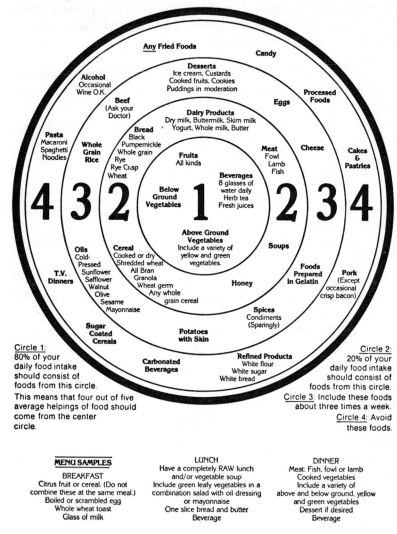

Circle 1:
80% of your daily food intake should consist of foods from this circle.

This means that four out of five average helpings of food should come from the center circle.

Circle 2:
20% of your daily food intake should consist of foods from this circle.

Circle 3: Include these foods about three times a week.

Circle 4: Avoid these foods.

MENU SAMPLES

BREAKFAST
Citrus fruit or cereal. (Do not combine these at the same meal.)
Boiled or scrambled egg
Whole wheat toast
Glass of milk

LUNCH
Have a completely RAW lunch and/or vegetable soup
Include green leafy vegetables in a combination salad with oil dressing or mayonnaise
One slice bread and butter
Beverage

DINNER
Meat: Fish, fowl or lamb
Cooked vegetables
Include a variety of above and below ground, yellow and green vegetables
Dessert if desired
Beverage

For the purpose of *losing* weight, only a few minor changes need to be made.

Circle 1—Stands as is except add potatoes.
Circle 2—Omit honey, whole milk, butter, granola. Add low-fat
        cheeses.
Circle 3—Move potatoes with skin to circle 1. Omit desserts,
        oils, puddings. Add raw sunflower seeds (dieters need
        the zinc).
Circle 4—Stands as is.

The following is representative of a typical day's intake for me. The fruits and vegetables change with the seasons. All foods are eaten raw, steamed, broiled, boiled, or microwaved, in that order.

See the Super-Dooper Pancake recipe on page 85, which I eat frequently instead of a regular meal. It's fast, simple, cheap, and nutritious. And non-fattening.

Bread is my binge food, therefore I don't eat bread. Period. So the wheat germ furnishes the needed B vitamins and unsaturated fats.

1000-CALORIE DAY

Food	Alkaline Calories	Acid Calories
Medium egg	65 (yolk)	15 (white)
Wheat germ, ½ cup		100
Banana or orange	100	
Broccoli—cup stalks	44	
Cottage cheese, ½ cup	90	
Tomato, 1 whole 2½"	30	
Baked potato	100	
Yellow squash—cup	34	
Lettuce—cup	15	
Spinach—cup	30	
Fish, fowl, lamb (measured portion)		100
Other dark greens— cup cooked	50 or less	
Pear—medium	80	
Yogurt, plain—cup	150	
Total=1003	788	215

While learning weight control, learn food selection based on nutrition, too.

Study the following basic nutrients list and select food that will provide some quantity of each nutrient daily. (Since science, medicine, and the health food folks do not agree on how much of each nutrient is needed by whom, allow your own consciousness to dictate how much *your* body requires.)

In the area of food selection, apply the knowledge you currently possess. More will be given as you come to know and understand better the workings of your own body. Each one of us has the responsibility for the maintenance of our health.

Remember that the body is subject to universal physical laws. However, circumstances alter cases. For example, medical conditions and physical conditions must be taken into consideration. Periods of stress increase the body's need for certain nutrients. Smokers require more vitamin C. Athletes may need slightly more protein.

Know Thyself!

BASIC NUTRIENTS AND THEIR SOURCES*

1. *Protein:* Fish, poultry, eggs, milk and cheese, dried beans (legumes), nuts and nut butters, wheat germ, brewers' yeast.

2. *Unsaturated fats:* Vegetable and most nut oils, salad dressings, mayonnaise, margarine, nuts and nut butters.

3. *Complex carbohydrates:* Flour and grain products, fruits, vegetables.

4. *Calcium:* Milk and milk products, dark green leafy vegetables, canned sardines and canned salmon, almonds, sesame seeds, soybeans, soy flour and soy products, oats, egg yolks.

5. *Iron:* Lean meats, glandular meats, chicken, especially dark meat; shellfish; dried beans (legumes); dried fruits, especially raisins, prunes and apricots; egg yolks; whole-grain products.

6. *Sodium:* Prepared foods, canned vegetables, meats, pickles, salt-water fish, milk, cheese, eggs, baking soda and baking powder, fresh carrots, beets, spinach, celery.

7. *Potassium:* Bananas; oranges; avocados; vegetables, particularly potatoes, winter squash, tomatoes, leafy greens.

8. *Magnesium:* Bananas, whole-grain products, dried beans (legumes), milk, dark green leafy vegetables, nuts.

9. *Phosphorous:* Whole-grain products, bran, cheese, milk, dried beans (legumes), eggs, meats, peanuts and peanut butter.

10. *Iodine:* Iodized and sea salt, kelp and other seaweed, saltwater seafoods.

11. *Zinc:* Beef, eggs, liver, herring, oyster, barley, brown rice, oatmeal, sunflower seeds, kelp and other seaweed, carrots, peas.

12. *Vitamin A:* Deep yellow and orange fruits and vegetables, especially carrots, sweet potatoes, apricots, winter squash, pumpkin and canteloupe; yellow corn and whole, unbolted yellow cornmeal; whole milk; cream; butter; whole-milk cheeses; liver; dark green vegetables, especially broccoli, escarole, spinach and parsley; tomatoes and tomato products.

---

*The Dieter's Companion: A Guide to Nutritional Self-Sufficiency, by Nikki and David Goldbeck, Signet, New York, 1977.

13. *Thiamine:* Pork, heart, kidneys, liver; dried beans (legumes), whole-grain products, wheat germ, brewers' yeast; nuts, especially peanuts and peanut butter.

14. *Riboflavin:* Meats, especially liver, kidneys and heart; milk and cheese; dark leafy greens; brewers' yeast; grain products.

15. *Niacin:* Lean meats, especially liver, poultry, fish; dried beans (legumes); whole-grain products; wheat germ; brewers' yeast; nuts, especially peanuts and peanut butter.

16. *Vitamin B-6:* Bananas, whole-grain products, chicken, dried beans (legumes), egg yolks, dark green leafy vegetables, fish and shellfish, meats, nuts, potatoes, prunes and raisins, brewers' yeast, wheat germ.

17. *Folacin:* Liver, dark green vegetables, dried beans (legumes), nuts.

18. *Pantothenic acid:* Organ meats, eggs, bran, peanuts, oats, whole wheat, wheat germ, pork, beef.

19. *Vitamin B-12:* Meats, particularly glandular meats, milk and cheese, fish, eggs and egg yolks, wheat germ, brewers' yeast, kelp and other seaweed.

20. *Vitamin C:* Fruits and vegetables, particularly citrus fruits, green and red pepper, tomatoes, potatoes cooked in their jackets, cantaloupe, strawberries, raw cabbage, brussels sprouts, broccoli.

21. *Vitamin D:* Fortified milk, egg yolks, fish-liver oils, sunshine.

22. *Vitamin E:* Vegetable oils, wheat germ and wheat germ oil, whole-grain products, peanuts, dark leafy greens.

HOW TO DESIGN YOUR OWN DIET
(What you will *normally* eat and drink
henceforth and forevermore!)

1. For medical reasons I do not/cannot/will not eat:

   _____

   _____

   _____

2. My favorite foods are: _____

   _____

   _____

   _____

3. I feel absolutely deprived if I do not eat occasionally:

   _____

   _____

   _____

4. My daily calorie limit will be _____

5. Alkaline calories _____ Acid calories _____

Keeping Eat Sheets

The reason for keeping records of what you are eating is the same as for counting calories—peace of mind.

Most of us are just too busy and preoccupied to remember if we ate "right," and that nagging doubt about did we overdo it or didn't we can be eliminated by writing down what we ate.

Also it is imperative to know that enough nutrients are being consumed to avoid future trouble. Always keep in mind that nourishment of cells is ongoing, and that those cells need something with which to build or else they will be weak.

Keep track of what you eat—at least temporarily—until you are sure that your nutritional bases are covered, and that you instinctively know which foods will keep your calorie count in line (and your waistline intact).

SUNDAY

	Alkaline Calories	Acid Calories
Breakfast		
Lunch		
Dinner		
Snacks		

TOTAL _____   TOTAL _____

74

MONDAY

	Alkaline Calories	Acid Calories
Breakfast	_____	_____
	_____	_____
	_____	_____
	_____	_____
Lunch	_____	_____
	_____	_____
	_____	_____
	_____	_____
Dinner	_____	_____
	_____	_____
	_____	_____
	_____	_____
Snacks	_____	_____
	_____	_____
	_____	_____
	_____	_____

TOTAL _____   TOTAL _____

TUESDAY

	Alkaline Calories	Acid Calories
Breakfast		
Lunch		
Dinner		
Snacks		
	TOTAL _____	TOTAL _____

WEDNESDAY

	Alkaline Calories	Acid Calories
Breakfast		
Lunch		
Dinner		
Snacks		

TOTAL _____   TOTAL _____

THURSDAY

	Alkaline Calories	Acid Calories
Breakfast		
Lunch		
Dinner		
Snacks		

TOTAL _____   TOTAL _____

FRIDAY

	Alkaline Calories	Acid Calories
Breakfast		
Lunch		
Dinner		
Snacks		
	TOTAL _____	TOTAL _____

SATURDAY

	Alkaline Calories	Acid Calories
Breakfast	_____	_____
	_____	_____
	_____	_____
	_____	_____
Lunch	_____	_____
	_____	_____
	_____	_____
	_____	_____
Dinner	_____	_____
	_____	_____
	_____	_____
	_____	_____
Snacks	_____	_____
	_____	_____
	_____	_____
	_____	_____

TOTAL _____   TOTAL _____

Behavior Modification

The following suggestions have proved to be of tremendous aid in altering conduct and habits that otherwise would prevent getting thin and staying thin.

Certain techniques appeal to some persons more than others. Best use can be made of them by including several at a time in the daily routine to determine which prove most helpful to you personally.

Consider them guidelines, not rules.

1. Always eat seated at a prettily set table, in a relaxed atmosphere; chew slowly.

2. While eating, think about how the food is renewing life and perpetuating health.

3. Welcome food as a favorite friend. Never treat any food as the enemy.

4. Try to allow enough time for meals so that you can stare at the last bite or two for five minutes. After that, if you still want it, eat it.

5. Notice if you feel regret when your plate is empty. Then permit yourself to choose to eat more. Then choose not to—for 20 minutes. If you are still hungry in a half hour, have something else so you can forget about food.

6. Use photos. The *before* will help to convince you how fat you are. The *after* will convince you how slim you are, which is just as hard to believe.

7. Pretend you are "on camera," and the whole world is watching you eat. Nobody ever stuffed down 22 cookies in front of an audience.

8. Tell yourself, "I don't think I can finish all this food." Then don't. You can sometimes fool yourself into thinking you are full when you aren't. The stomach will obey—eventually—because "mind is the builder."

9. Think small: small dishes, small portions, small clothes, mini-goals.

10. Think green. To lose weight and stay healthy, we have to eat raw, green veggies. We don't have to like them, we just have to eat them.

11. Keep quiet about your diet. If you don't, someone inevitably will try to talk you out of it. This time instead of talking, do something.

12. Get enough sleep. Dieting causes stress, which will overcome all

efforts. Stress causes the body's survival mechanism to trigger. Then wild horses couldn't stop us from eating. Sufficient rest will convince our bodies that we really aren't trying to starve to death. Eventually the body relaxes and begins to cooperate with what the mind is telling it to do. It then gets easier.

13. Guard against cumulative hunger. Eating too little will always backfire. Hunger sneaks up, compelling us to gorge on whatever is handy.

14. Avoid your binge foods. For some eating NO bread is easier than stopping with 1 slice. And what true ice-cream freak ever stopped with a meager half cup?

15. Look for spiritual help. All knowledge is within. It becomes available when the God within is aligned with the God without. But your inner guidance may direct you to a commercial weight-control program. If it does—go.

16. Acknowledge yourself and allow yourself to change. You are not only a body but a mind and a soul, too. Each of these three aspects that make up the self is intensely interested in what you are attempting to do.

17. Fear nothing. Not even success. Once you get spiritual help into the act, transformative powers are loosed within, which may shake your life to its foundations. It then takes courage to continue.

18. Recognize that others perceive you differently when you are thin than when you are fat. The resulting anxieties can usually be overcome with patience.

19. Believe in the rightness of your efforts. Taking the time to assure your nutritional and caloric needs is not selfish. If being overweight is sapping your strength and/or draining you mentally, then it is more selfish to stay fat. Once you begin recording your caloric and nutritional intake, you can forget about it and yourself. You then will be free to do for and think about others, which is the key to happiness.

20. Hold realistic expectations. Solving your weight problem will make your doctor happy. Other than that, the only dilemma losing weight will do is to release you from the repression caused by being fat. Then you can focus your energies on other important situations.

21. Keep your perspective. Attitude is everything. Rather than feel deprived because you are giving up non-nutritive foods, feel happy that you are doing something for yourself that you know will pay off.

22. Love yourself. The world needs what you have to offer. Appreciate the uniqueness of what it means to be you—and stop hiding. Even though "much is asked of those who are aware," the challenge is exhilarating.

Dreams

The Edgar Cayce readings say that anything of any importance that happens to us is first previewed in our dreams.

There were two remarkable dreams that positively affected my efforts to lose weight. Unfortunately, I have a bad habit of omitting the year from the date in my journals, so I can't be sure of the year. I believe, though, the first dream presented itself in 1973:

The entire dream consisted of a large, black woman, who asked, "Why does being fat matter?"

I answered, "It doesn't matter if it doesn't matter!" *End.*

The woman's question and my answer to her surprised me at first. Consciously I must have been under the impression that being overweight was *always* a cause for concern. Then pondering the question, I concluded that, indeed, being fat does not matter if the excess weight does not hinder one's purpose in the earth, which for all of us, whether we believe it or not, is to learn to love through fulfilling our potential as co-creators with the Father.

The second dream occurred a year or so later during a difficult period when I couldn't seem to stick to a sensible eating plan and, of course, the weight loss had stopped. I was discouraged, if not defeated. This dream demonstrated that not only did it matter to me, but that I would win. It was like a vision:

I, a 200-pound Linda, was watching a 200-pound Linda watch a 135-pound Linda riding toward "us" astride a magnificent white stallion. The "future" Linda was wearing a Grecian robe, complete with gold braids and "her" hair was full and loosely curled around her face. "Our" hair, at the time, was shorter and straighter. As the stallion approached us, he reared up on his hind legs, and we were astonished to see the words, "Victory! Victory!" appear in the air above them. *End.*

For days afterward I was so happy I felt as it I were floating, enchanted by the image the dream presented. I knew that someday I would somehow emerge victorious and in control of all the aspects of self that the dream presented.

A third dream occurred only this year. At the time, I was craving sweets but fighting it. In the dream I was given this recipe:

Dream Cookies

Only the ingredients were given with the explicit instructions that three raisins were to top each cookie.

Ingredients:	Calories:
6 egg whites, beaten into meringue	102
1 cup raw wheat germ	412
½ teaspoon almond flavoring	negligible
½ teaspoon cinnamon	negligible
6 envelopes Sweet and Low®	negligible
Raisins, 3 tablespoons	40

The dream left it up to me to figure out the rest:

Fold the wheat germ and seasonings carefully into the egg whites. Drop by the teaspoonful onto a non-stick baking sheet. Carefully place three raisins atop each cookie. (I realized later that the raisins, while delightfully symbolic of the Trinity, also nicely remove the aftertaste left by the Sweet and Low®.)

Bake at 325° for half an hour or until nicely browned.

Makes 64 cookies at fewer than nine calories each!

The basic recipe adapts nicely to a substitute for torte.

Dream Torte

Prepare an eight- or nine-inch pie pan by spraying a nonstick substance or by buttering *very* lightly. (Butter should be used in any recipe as if one stick had to last a year.)

"Crust":

¼ cup raw sunflower seeds sprinkled in the bottom of the pie pan.

Filling:

Pour the egg white/wheat germ/seasonings mixture on top of the sunflower seeds. Sprinkle the top with the raisins. Bake at 300° for half an hour or until browned.

Serves eight persons at 95 calories per slice.

For a very special treat, serve the torte or cookies with a delicious substitute for cream cheese. It's so delicious, I've named it Dream Cheese. . .

Dream Cheese
   Ingredients:
   Part skim milk ricotta cheese
   Low-fat cottage cheese
   To prepare, mix half ricotta and half cottage cheese together with a food processor (it's too heavy for a blender). Sprinkle with butter-flavored popcorn salt to taste. One-half cup contains only 120 calories versus 100 calories for one mere ounce of cream cheese. (And even my kids can't tell the difference.)

Linda's Super-Dooper Power-Packed Pancakes

Ingredients:	Calories:
1 egg	80
¼ cup wheat germ (raw)	100
Heaping tablespoon raw sunflower seeds	90

Stir together egg and wheat germ. Add water as necessary to obtain desired consistency. (It should be pourable.) Pour into non-stick skillet. Sprinkle with raw sunflower seeds. Cook 5 minutes on one side. Turn and cook until the sunflower seeds are nicely browned and the pancake is done throughout.

This pancake provides protein, unsaturated fats, carbohydrates, calcium, iron, sodium, magnesium, phosphorous, zinc, thiamin, riboflavin, niacin, B-6, folacin, pantothenic acid, B-12, D, and E.

A light sprinkling of sea salt or Morton's Lite salt provides iodine.

Pancake Topping
   1 mashed banana
   Provides potassium, some C, more magnesium.

That's some quantity of 21 of the 22 basic nutrients. Another meal made of tomatoes, carrots, and green vegetables provides Vitamin A plus reinforcements of other needed nutrients—plenty of power for very few calories!

Exercise

Which exercises are most effective? The ones we do. And do. And do.

Again, it's a matter of consciousness. While some walk, others must run. What really counts is that the activity be fun and/or gratifying, else we won't keep on keeping on. Persistence is the key.

St. Francis of Assisi is reported to have referred to his body as "Brother Ass." I suspect that this is because of his difficulty in getting his body to cooperate with his mind and spirit. I have the same problem.

A personal observation about the body as related to exercise: The body can't be trusted. Contrary to the opinion of many experts, ol' buddy Body is highly unreliable as a judge of what it needs. The body is only the result of what has been built with the mind. If mind has been busily creating on its own, without benefit of guidance from the Source, Body may be in big trouble.

Body is subject to physical laws. Just because mind has aligned with spirit and is now reconstructing and remodeling the temple, it may take a while for Body to catch up.

However, Body can be coaxed along, nurtured and encouraged, until finally one grand day, it will respond to the new conditioning mind has been giving it and will begin to shape up (no pun intended) on its own. No amount of spiritual and mental work will transform a fat, flabby, weak body. Physical conditions require physical healings. In 1936 a 57-year-old woman requested: "Please advise how I may *through meditation* rejuvenate my body." Cayce answered:

Rejuvenate the physical first! Then we may make a better accord for the mental and the spiritual to be active through same!

So seldom is it considered by all, that spirituality, mentality, and the physical being are all one; yet may indeed separate and function one without the other—and *one at the expense of the other* [emphasis mine].

Make them cooperative, make them one in their purpose—and we will have a greater activity.   **307-10**

This reading explains to me why in our Western civilization many beautiful spirits are physically out of condition. We would do well to remember that the human race is governed by spiritual, mental AND *physical* laws:

Do the first things first. Lay the stress on those things that are necessary [eating right and exercising]. Remember, healing—all healing—comes from within. Yet there is the healing of the physical, there is the healing of the mental, there is the correct direction from the spirit. Coordinate these and you'll be whole! *But to attempt to do a physical healing through the mental conditions is the misdirection of the spirit that prompts same—* **the same that brings about accidents, the same that brings about the eventual separation. For it is** *law.* **But when the law is coordinated, in spirit, in mind, in** *body,* **the entity is capable of fulfilling the purpose for which it enters a material or physical experience.**

Do that. . .

Keep in those ways in which there is the putting of the stress upon that needed, see? not attempting to use spiritual forces in the place of mental attitudes, nor use mental attitudes in the place of material adjustments; but coordinating same one to another.   **2528-2**

A Word of Caution About Fasting

Many people get so desperate about losing weight and become so frustrated with attempting to *choose* foods, they give up eating altogether—for a few days.

While fasting for 24-36 hours for cleansing is safe enough for most, longer periods without food in the hope of losing weight is nothing more than a diverson, a trick we play on ourselves to postpone the inevitable learning that must occur if we are to develop freedom of choice.

Fasting for the purpose of losing weight can provide a temporary reprieve to those tormented by battling with food, but it is useless and even destructive over the long haul.

Not eating only postpones the ability to choose.

Weight control is entirely dependent upon *choices*. Not eating anything at all is infinitely easier—temporarily—than eating limited amounts. Enough willpower can be mustered to do anything for a day or two. But choices are not dependent on willpower; they depend on purpose, motivation, the ideal, the "why bother" behind one's decisions.

Perhaps the most important point of all to be made about fasting is this: Cellular re-creation is never-ceasing. And during times of self-deprivation the cells are building with inferior materials. The nutrients available are inferior, and, most of all, the *thoughts* with which the cells re-create are inferior because they are thoughts of *self-delusion*.

During periods of fasting, the metabolism slows down. The body, having a consciousness of its own and separate from the mind with which you "think," will fight to maintain the status quo, to retain its mass. This lack of "oneness"—this separation of mind, body, and spirit—is the cause of weight problems, food problems, physical problems, etc., in the first place. Learning to choose builds cooperation between body and mind that is guided by spirit.

To deprive the cells of the body of nutrients and creative, self-actualizing thoughts perpetuates and actually encourages aging, dis-ease, and slow death.

So as not to end on that depressing note, let me add that choosing to fast for a day or so can be undertaken harmlessly by holding constantly the thoughts that the body is resting, rejuvenating and re-creating itself into a more pleasing thought form. For, indeed, our bodies are precisely that. . .*thought forms*.

Journal Work

It is believed by some that the number 28 contains the consciousness of God and God alone directing. It has been suggested that anything that is done for 28 days consecutively becomes a habit.

A study of The Revelation in the Bible, aided by *A Commentary on the Book of the Revelation,** reveals the symbology of the numbers 7 and 4, which multiplied equal 28. Adding 2 to 8 equals 10 which, in numerology, equals 1—the symbolic number of the one true God.

The following pages contain the self-image-building journal. There is one page for each of 28 days. Daily affirmation of the self as a co-creator, an extension of the Father's reality, reinforces the belief in your ability to accomplish any task. It is designed to be used in conjunction with meditation to establish daily the inner-life connection so vital to success.

Give yourself time each day to do this journal work because you deserve it. Treat yourself also to a copy of *Day by Day,*** compiled by Dee Shambaugh and Herbert Bruce Puryear, also published by A.R.E. Press. *Day by Day* is the perfect partner in the image building and disciplinary work necessary to accomplish a major transformation, be it in your weight or any other area of your life.

**A Commentary on the Book of the Revelation,* by the Association for Research and Enlightenment, A.R.E. Press, Virginia Beach, Va., 1969.
***Day by Day: Steps to a New Life,* by Dolores Shambaugh and Herbert B. Puryear, Ph.D., A.R.E. Press, Virginia Beach, Va., 1981.

Day 1

Patience

Patience is the art of accepting, while transforming, reality.

We get discouraged when trying to reach a goal because we want everything to happen easily and quickly—immediately would be nice.

We become so dismayed by our inadequacies—real or imagined—that we give up. Before we know it, life has passed us by.

We must start from where we are because here is where we are. And here is where we shall stay until we move into some other place in consciousness.

Complete the following:
Today I celebrate my new beginning by _____

_____

_____

_____

_____

_____

_____

_____

_____

_____

_____

Visualization

Visualization is the art of calling to mind images of what you would become. Manifestation of these images is inevitable. It is the Law.

During moments of concentrated imagery, the cells are re-creating with the consciousness of that held in the mind. This, too, is Law. Use it wisely.

Complete the following:
Today I see myself _____

_____

_____

_____

_____

_____

_____

_____

_____

_____

_____

_____

_____

Mind

Mind is the builder, the creator, or the co-creator. Depending on our purpose, we build and create in and of ourselves, or we tap into the Source and co-create far beyond what we could manage alone.

Limitless potential is our inherent right.

Complete the following:

Today my mind builds a bridge on which I safely cross the whirlpool of ego, the rapids of anger, the currents of fear and injustice. My bridge is being built with qualities of _____

_____

_____

_____

_____

_____

_____

_____

_____

_____

_____

_____

Creation

"Creation has been defined as being recognizable by the intensity of the encounter.

"What is this encounter with?"*

As it relates to weight control, the encounter will always be with attitudes and emotions that are held in consciousness by the very cells themselves.

But cellular consciousness can be changed as can the identity of any creation, if it is only returned into the hands of the original Creator. Cooperation with the original Artist hastens change.

Complete the following:

Today I commit myself to the creative process going on within my cells, my soul, my mind by ————

———————————————————————

———————————————————————

———————————————————————

———————————————————————

———————————————————————

———————————————————————

———————————————————————

———————————————————————

———————————————————————

*The Courage to Create, by Rollo May, Bantam Books, New York, N.Y., 1980.

93

Relationships

Relationships depend on the way we treat others. So how can we be considerate, responsive, and concerned for the welfare of others, yet at the same time be immune to what they think? It is illogical. Nobody lives in a vacuum.

But being aware of divergent opinions is not the same as being dependent on those opinions, which may be untrue or obsolete.

Complete the following:

Today I am a color in the rainbow of brotherhood, blending in perfect harmony with all whom I meet.

My color is _____ because I feel

_____

_____

_____

_____

_____

_____

_____

_____

_____

_____

Response-Ability

Response-ability, like responsibility, develops with maturity. Our ability to respond to new persons and situations, and the willingness to make new commitments, increase as our self-image improves.

To answer the call within us and to accept being held accountable denote qualities of the highest calling.

Complete the following:

Today I am a mountain climber. An irresistible challenge compels me to scale the highest pinnacle of my life, which is _____

_____

_____

_____

_____

_____

_____

_____

_____

_____

_____

Achievement

Achievement is as basic to the human heart as is the need to be acknowledged. It is fully as real as the body's need for food, and it can be equally as satisfying. This by no means implies one must rush around doing things to justify one's existence. Rather view achievement as something as simple, yet complex—to say nothing of important—as learning to cope with food.

We tend to measure our self-esteem by what we do. Everyone needs a place to shine a little. This can be your finest hour.

Complete the following:
To date, my most satisfying achievement has been

_____

_____

_____

_____

_____

_____

_____

_____

_____

Vibration

Vibration is life. Like music, the entire universe is in constant, vibrating motion. It flows, changes, turns, ebbs, evolves, spirals, circles, expands, contracts.

To touch this vibration, to feel one's own body in harmony with all creation, is an evolutionary experience worth waiting and working for.

Foods, too, are vibration. To sense these vibrations and become attuned to the life within foods is to be able to gauge one's own inner development. The body is built with the vibrations of the foods one eats.

Choose life!

Complete the following:

Today I am a musical instrument playing my part in life's symphony. I am a _____ because I feel

_____

_____

_____

_____

_____

_____

_____

_____

_____

Confidence

By acquiring confidence in your abilities, you can discover untapped excellence within yourself.

You need not fear overreaching your capacities, but you must not undervalue and underemploy them.

You are a complex creature, capable of great despair, but also of great delight.

Confidence in yourself is delight in being who you are, in what you are becoming, in discovering the endless, though sometimes exasperating adventure of what it means to be you.

Complete the following:

Today I am the sea. I see only my surface, but I feel my depths, my power, my richness. My hidden treasures are _____

_____

_____

_____

_____

_____

_____

_____

_____

_____

Mistakes

Mistakes are to be treasured as your most precious allies. Victory is not always at hand. Indeed, it is through apparent failures that the strongest quality in humanity—the refusal to stay defeated—grows stronger.

Being consistently, persistently, stubbornly cheerful allows us to choose what will be done with mistakes.

Complete the following:

Today I close the door on the past and open the door to a future filled with _____

_____

_____

_____

_____

_____

_____

_____

_____

_____

_____

_____

Day 11 **Flexibility**

Flexibility is the ability not to be thrown for a loop by the unexpected.

When circumstances turn your most carefully made plans inside out, flow with them. Pause and regroup—think, don't react. Then do whatever you have to do.

You will discover powers within yourself as yet unsuspected and possibilities as yet undreamed of.

Complete the following:
Today I am fire imparting warmth and light to all who come into my glow. My fuel is the understanding of

_____

_____

_____

_____

_____

_____

_____

_____

_____

_____

_____

Rules can often be a guide for successful living, but they are no substitute for living. Rules can never quite keep up· with reality because rules come from experience, not vice versa.

Life happens. And being infinitely inventive, it will always outrun and outmaneuver any attempt to bottle it up in a cut-and-dried system.

Complete the following:
Today I will tear down fences I have built around myself. Fences of rules, fears, worries, anxieties all will be gone when I _____

_____

_____

_____

_____

_____

_____

_____

_____

_____

_____

Direction

Direction depends on our purpose for being in the earth.

Sometimes we forget our purpose and get lost. Then we backtrack and begin again. We may still be lost, but we may have learned which way *not* to go.

Remember *Alice in Wonderland:*

Alice: "Oh, Puss, which way shall I go?"

Puss: "That depends a great deal on where you want to get to."

Alice: "Oh, I don't care much where."

Puss: "Then it doesn't much matter which way you go."

Complete the following:

Today light illuminates my purpose and purpose directs my path to ⎯⎯⎯⎯⎯⎯⎯⎯

⎯⎯⎯⎯⎯⎯⎯⎯⎯⎯⎯⎯⎯⎯⎯⎯

⎯⎯⎯⎯⎯⎯⎯⎯⎯⎯⎯⎯⎯⎯⎯⎯

⎯⎯⎯⎯⎯⎯⎯⎯⎯⎯⎯⎯⎯⎯⎯⎯

⎯⎯⎯⎯⎯⎯⎯⎯⎯⎯⎯⎯⎯⎯⎯⎯

⎯⎯⎯⎯⎯⎯⎯⎯⎯⎯⎯⎯⎯⎯⎯⎯

⎯⎯⎯⎯⎯⎯⎯⎯⎯⎯⎯⎯⎯⎯⎯⎯

⎯⎯⎯⎯⎯⎯⎯⎯⎯⎯⎯⎯⎯⎯⎯⎯

⎯⎯⎯⎯⎯⎯⎯⎯⎯⎯⎯⎯⎯⎯⎯⎯

Happiness

Happiness is the state or quality of being pleased or content. Pleasure felt during the attempt to construct a new creation energizes the determination to see the project through to completion.

Complete the following:
Today my greatest source of happiness is _____

_____

_____

_____

_____

_____

_____

_____

_____

_____

_____

_____

_____

_____

Willpower

Willpower fades into oblivion when replaced with purpose.

Having a purpose for any accomplishment guarantees achievements far surpassing anything that can be reached through mere willpower.

True, conscious choices are made through use of the will, but inner strength developed through motivation and purpose creates a permanent change in attitude toward ourselves, food, our bodies, or our fellow humans.

Complete the following:
Today my motivation and purpose are _____

_____

_____

_____

_____

_____

_____

_____

_____

_____

_____

Dis-ease

Dis-ease and disharmony may threaten to strike the body when the mind attempts to regain control over the physical.

Having a consciousness of its own, the physical body may attempt to rebel at changes in the status quo, at relinquishing control to the mind that is being guided by spirit.

The conscious mind remains open to the suggestion that "you must eat or you may get sick."

Accepting this suggestion means that, once again, flesh will win out over spirit.

Resistance to the threat of dis-ease is strengthened through sufficient and balanced nutrition, adequate exercise, and through getting enough rest.

Complete the following:
Today my thoughts weave a tapestry of healing tranquillity and loving service. I can best serve others as well as myself by doing ――――――――――

――――――――――――――――――――

――――――――――――――――――――

――――――――――――――――――――

――――――――――――――――――――

――――――――――――――――――――

――――――――――――――――――――

――――――――――――――――――――

――――――――――――――――――――

Nature is cyclical, as are we humans. The ocean's tides rise and fall, yet we do not view low tide as a weakness of the sea.

Roses do not bloom all year round, but when they do, we possess the wisdom to allow the natural process to bring the rose to maturity. We instinctively know that ripping the petals apart may open the rose but will destroy it in the process.

Every choice that we make throughout the day moves us toward or away from the beauty of a healthy, mature rose. Through wise choices we may bring great joy and loveliness into the lives of many, if we have the patience to wait gently on ourselves—and prepare not to miss the brief moment of maturity.

Grieve not for missed moments, however, for they shall return as surely as the next high tide.

Complete the following:
Today I am as a rosebud. I resist not my unfoldment into a masterful creation which will be completed when

_____

_____

_____

_____

_____

_____

_____

_____

Belief Day 18

Believe in yourself. In a world of carbon-copy look-a-likes, you are distinct.

Your sensitivity, talents, and tastes are unparalleled. If you do not value and use them, they will be wasted. No one else has your particular combination of abilities.

You are needed.

Complete the following:
Today I shall overcome my disbelief in _____

_____

_____

_____

_____

_____

_____

_____

_____

_____

_____

_____

_____

107

Day 19 **Practice**

Practicing what you hope to become is neither phoniness nor pretension.

Athletes, artists, and musicians practice techniques and skills to polish, hone, and refine their work.

Weight-control skills are learnable, and with practice they become a part of the whole person.

Practice looking beautiful. There is nothing shameful about putting forth your best any more than there is about painting your house and mowing the lawn.

Because you are so special and appealing, it is more fraudulent not to be as attractive as you can. To be less is to cheat the world and yourself.

The manner in which we present ourselves to others reflects who we are within.

Complete the following:
Today I will practice becoming outwardly all that I am inwardly. I am intelligent, talented and _____

_____

_____

_____

_____

_____

_____

_____

Knowledge

Knowledge without application is pathetic.

Knowing *about* life does not imply living any more than knowing *about* weight loss implies success.

One's capacity for *doing* enlarges by *doing*.

Only then does *knowing* become meaningful.

Complete the following:

Today I am a student learning to _____

_____

_____

_____

_____

_____

_____

_____

_____

_____

_____

_____

Desire

Desires are qualities of the spirit within.

The desire to conquer the physical is but a remembrance of our inheritance of eternal life. Many desires are the soul's demands for its own fulfillment.

The desire to be thin does not lessen with age. Whatever your present age, you will desire a slim, healthy vehicle for the soul no less ten or twenty years from now.

Why waste the intervening years?

Complete the following:

Today my desire for undesirable foods is replaced with a desire for _____

_____

_____

_____

_____

_____

_____

_____

_____

_____

_____

Beauty is a noble pursuit. Consider this from the Edgar Cayce readings:

Thus prepare thy body, prepare thy way. For there is nothing in heaven or hell that may separate the soul from the Maker save self. He, thy Father-God, will not withhold any good thing from those who love His coming. Thy body is indeed the temple of the living God. There He has promised to meet thee often. Meet Him, in joy, in song, in prayer. Thus ye will find thy life blossoming—physically, mentally and spiritually— even as the rose. And the very fragrance of thy life, the beauty of thy life, will make and bring joy to many. This is as little as ye can give for the great gift of beauty ye make in the lives of others. 3440-2

Complete the following:
Today the world is more beautiful because I am here because _____

_____

_____

_____

_____

_____

_____

_____

_____

Consistency

Consistency in our actions will close the credibility gap between the conscious and the unconscious minds.

When we say, for instance, that we want to gain control over our physical body, but then act out contradictions to that stated idea, the unconscious mind refuses to take our efforts seriously.

On the other hand, when we behave in accordance with our stated desires, the unconscious mind will eventually begin to believe us and to cooperate.

We then begin to make correct food choices automatically, without conflict.

Complete the following:
Today I will consistently _____

_____

_____

_____

_____

_____

_____

_____

_____

_____

_____

_____

_____

_____

_____

Persistence

Persistence practically *guarantees* success.

It is worth noting that Thomas Edison tried *six thousand* substances before he found the one that would work as a filament in his light bulb.

Babe Ruth struck out more times than any other baseball player in history.

Apparent failure is the common denominator among many, but persistence is what sets the achievers apart from the others.

Complete the following:
Today I will persistently _____

_____

_____

_____

_____

_____

_____

_____

_____

_____

_____

_____

_____

_____

_____

_____

Rewards

Rewards of being slim will vary from time to time. Occasionally, doubt will creep in causing you to wonder if there are rewards involved at all.

Self-pity may emerge as the primary emotion at these times, but rest assured, these times are always temporary.

Complete the following:

Today I reward myself for having the intelligence to short-circuit the "poor-deprived-me" syndrome with

_____

_____

_____

_____

_____

_____

_____

_____

_____

_____

_____

_____

_____

_____

_____

_____

Initiation into the society of the transformed few began the moment when desire entered the mind.

Membership is assured when that desire is allowed its life. It will direct you through the necessary steps and will never fail you.

Complete the following:
Today my desire to be slender will be given full rein. I will _____

_____

_____

_____

_____

_____

_____

_____

_____

_____

_____

_____

_____

_____

_____

_____

_____

_____

Transitions

Transition, the act of passing from one place or condition to another, requires understanding that others' perceptions may change as we do.

Certain expectations remain constant, and it takes patience to allow others to catch up with where we are.

Complete the following:
Today I am aware of changes in _____

_____

_____

_____

_____

_____

_____

_____

_____

_____

_____

_____

_____

_____

_____

_____

_____

Perfection

Perfection of the physical body, like art, is subjective. Not all desire to live within identical forms.

Consider the following from Gina Cerminara's *The World Within* *'on the necessity of perfection of the physical body:

". . .any deviation from harmony or proportion or health is indicative of some psychic necessity somewhere." (p. 51)

". . .all of us, men and women alike, can be prompted by the long-range view of many lifetimes, to the awareness of our own obligation to strive consciously for beauty, on all levels of being.

"This must be done almost impersonally, however, and without sensual attachment; in the spirit, as (Edgar) Cayce puts it, of 'making a perfect sacrifice, holy, acceptable unto God.' It must be done with the same sort of terrible compulsion that an artist feels to transfer some beautiful image to canvas, or a sculptor to capture some lovely proportions in stone. For unless it is done out of such an impersonal passion for beauty itself, and out of a kind of sense of obligation to render to the universe a gift at least as beautiful as the most insignificant of nature's handiwork, the beautiful body we create will become itself a terrible snare, trap, and delusion." (pp. 80-81)

*The World Within, by Gina Cerminara, Ph.D., William Sloane Associates, New York City, N.Y., 1957.

Complete the following:

Today, at the end of this 28-day cycle, as I consider what "perfection" means to me, I review my choices. I perceive them to be _____

_____

_____

_____

_____

_____

_____

_____

_____

_____

_____

_____

_____

_____

_____

_____

_____

_____

_____

_____

_____

_____

Auto-Suggestion

The subconscious mind has been described as the garbage dump where all manner of rotting ideas linger. Not a very pretty picture to be sure, but accurate.

These old ideas block the connection between the conscious mind where we make conscious decisions, and the unconscious where knowledge is perfect and application is automatic.

To bring this ability to know and apply into consciousness (to get it up front where we can work with it), it is necessary to clear a path so the part of us that remembers itself to be perfect can get through.

A 65-year-old woman asked Edgar Cayce in 1931:

Q-3. Any spiritual advice for this body?
A-3. The body is spiritual in its aspects and in its reaction. If the body will aid self in those applications as may be made for same, see self—in the periods when the body enters into the quiet—healed as it, the body, would be healed. Vision self being aided by those applications. Know what each application is for, seeing that doing that within self. Keep the mind in that attitude as makes for continuity of forces manifesting through self—a continual flow, see?   **326-1**

Within each of us lives an idea, a thought form that meets the standards of perfection originally intended by our Creator. But somewhere along the way, we co-creators had ideas of our own; and, thinking that we knew better, we botched ourselves up. At this moment, we are manifesting the results of the thoughts and ideas that replaced the original intention.

But fortunately, the memory of ourselves as we were—as we are, if we but believe it—is alive and well within us, but hiding behind a maze of psychological blocks we have built into our physical consciousness. Finding our way through this maze could take forever if we depend on our conscious resources only. But we have unconscious resources, a method of clearing a path, breaking down the blocks, unraveling the maze. We can be free of entanglement with perplexity, uncertainty, and bewilderment.

We can be free of self-created fears, doubt, confusion about truth and, most of all, free of our emotional involvement with food.

Scientists and metaphysicians agree that there is a space between being awake and being asleep called *twilight*. During this twilight state, the conscious and unconscious minds are susceptible to suggestion. While in this yielding, open state, the subconscious part of the mind where the negatives live (and work their mischief) apparently is less resistant to change and cleansing. It is during this twilight state that we can make our greatest breakthroughs in bringing into consciousness our ideals. We can receive true cooperation from the "higher self" and shorten the time required to manifest a different thought form, truly, a different body.

The use of suggestion during the twilight state is in addition to visualization during waking hours. What we *hold* in the mind will manifest. But auto-suggestion differs from imaging in that visualization is a creating, a conjuring of images, pictures, visions of how we would like to look. Auto-suggestion is the pouring in, the introduction into the subconscious, of new seeds which will push roots through the subconscious until they tap into the source of life and begin to blossom forth on their own. These newly planted seeds, new thoughts, will find their way through the negatives which seek to block their path.

As in nature, these new seeds must be helped along, reinforced and protected until such time that they can thrive alone. In this case, consciously choosing to eat the right foods and participating in some form of exercise is the same as watering and fertilizing newly planted seeds.

To begin, you need equipment: Tape recorder, blank tape, written suggestion which you will read into the tape. (The sound of your own voice strikes a more responsive chord within than that of another's voice.)

Words that work: The following is only a suggested format. You may add or subtract as you wish. Only *you* know how your mind will react to any given wording. If you care to be more specific, such as using your name, height, weight, by all means do so. In that case you would begin. . .

My name is _____

I am _____ tall and my weight is _____ pounds

(ideal)

(. . .then move into. . .)

I am a creator. I am creating
a perfect temple wherein truth and
beauty dwell.

My weight is perfect for my height.

I am a light
unto my world.

My bearing is erect and proud.

My thoughts are healing
to myself and others.

I am serene within myself,
a perfect channel.

Each night while falling asleep, play the tape on which you have repeated the suggestion at least ten times. You don't wish to be interrupted by having to replay the tape. Obviously, a recorder with an automatic shutoff is convenient, but not necessary.

While listening to the recording, relax into the words and trust the Universal Law to assure their effectiveness.

It might help to remember, "In the beginning was the Word. . ." Also, words are what separates us from lower forms of life. Words have their own vibration and must be spoken aloud or written to have their life.

Use this space to write your suggestion:

_____

_____

_____

_____

Level Six

"I Have Done It!"
(Now what?)

Free at last
Thin at last
All my problems
Are in the past—
Or are they?

I have some good news. . .you're skinny!

And some bad news. . .your work has just begun.

For one thing, you may not be satisfied with the way your body looks or feels.

In a world where bodies are supposed to be beautiful, you may look at yours and decide that even if it isn't fat, it isn't exactly beautiful. A sag here, a leftover lump there, well, it can be downright discouraging. So discouraging, in fact, that still not liking one's body after all that work is one reason so many regain all the weight. They figure it just isn't worth it. They still can't wear some of the clothes they would enjoy, and being seen *out* of one's clothes remains unthinkable.

It's all a matter of perspective.

For myself, it took 39 years to realize that the producer of *Charlie's Angels* was not going to call no matter how skinny I was. But it's okay because I'm in control of my body and my life.

Our bodies are thought forms. However, it may take as many lifetimes to rebuild ourselves into what we think we *want* to be as it has to become what we *are*. And being simply *not fat* is a good beginning. The physical habits and psychological reshuffling that have brought us to this point where we are not fat must continue for the rest of our lives.

Remaining in our bodies are cells which hold the consciousness of being fat. These cells will continue to struggle to have their life. Sending signals to the brain, these cells demand food. It takes, for some, years of experience to detect these signals and interrupt them before the brain accepts them and demands excessive food.

A most helpful method of fighting this battle is to continue meditating in the knowledge that the cells which are re-creating during the moments of meditation will live and reproduce within your body, crowding out the cells which do not agree with your ideal. Meditation also will help you to continue to exercise and choose foods wisely. But weight won't meditate away.

To *get* the weight off you ate the right foods and exercised.

To *keep* the weight off you learn to *like* eating the right foods— and exercise.

The best thing that could possibly happen to you now is to wake up one morning craving celery and pears. If you were to all of a sudden adore plain raw veggies, and if your idea of a ducky good time were to do a couple of hours of snappy calesthenics, and if the moon were made of green cheese. . .

I'm not saying it won't happen. That would be negative programming. But the facts are that only one in 17 people who lose weight *never* regain an ounce. (And I'm betting that one is a tall man with a hyperactive thyroid.)

However, you not only *can* keep *most* of it off *all* of the time, you *will* keep *all* of it off *most* of the time. Losers are winners, but regainers are losers. From here on out, the best days of your life will be those days when you have nothing left to lose!

Keeping the weight off is easy—sometimes.

When life is exciting, the work's going well, nobody is sick, money is plentiful, and there's something fun to look forward to, nutritious, non-fattening food choices are almost automatic. Savor these times as the blessings they are. But don't fall into a sense of false security.

124

"The Poem"

If life were but a joyful high where I just soared
    and touched the sky,
I'd never think of pie.
But life's down here where all's hard sell, and
    I'm just muddling through the hell,
And chocolate chips are swell.
When I'm not bored but busily attending to the
    needs I see,
I sip only plain tea.
As often, though, my worldly cares are met
    with blank, unfeeling stares,
But not from the eclairs.

Life moves in cycles and seasons. Everything is not perfect every minute of every day of your life. (If it were, you couldn't stand it.) So be prepared.

Keep the refrigerator stocked with foods that you can eat. No matter what else happens, don't run out of your foods and be forced by circumstances to eat any old thing that's handy. When you suddenly increase your intake of sugars and empty carbohydrates such as those in processed foods, your body can't handle them.

Almost everyone agrees that eating junk food leaves you hungry. So now you have stress and abnormal hunger to deal with, and all of it together can be just too much. If you feed the stress and the hunger, you are well on your way to proving out the statistics.

When your guard goes down, the scale goes up. Scales should come equipped with a little red flag that pops up at the three-pound-over-goal number. Or a talking sign that jumps up and shouts, "This way to Fat City." Then maybe it wouldn't take so long to get right back to the habits that led to success. And get back to those habits you must, so the sooner the better.

Remember that a temporary relapse isn't the end of the world. You're too smart to try to fool yourself into believing that you can ever go back to mindless eating without gaining weight. If you binge on weekends, on Monday mornings you'll be overweight by maybe as much as seven or eight pounds.

Ann, a 39-year-old, five-foot-ten, blond amazon with 34-inch hips, says she regains the same seven pounds every weekend. The weight she gains from Friday night till Sunday night takes her from Monday to the following Friday to lose. But lose it she does. It's a way of life for her that enables her to socialize, yet remain slender and, even more important, in control of herself.

It helps to hang out with and emulate naturally thin people. Mickey, an over-40 size 8, who's never been five pounds overweight in her life, nibbles her food. That girl can make half a sandwich last 30 minutes. Her whole consciousness is tiny. She takes tiny bites, tiny steps, even her voice is tiny. So is her waist.

Marie, age 60, five-foot-six, whose weight in her entire life except when pregnant never topped 135 pounds, takes time out to eat—always. She says that no matter what else is going on she must eat three meals a day, beginning with a hot breakfast. She also says that eating proper meals is the most important part of her day. There's a lesson there for the rest of us.

If you should happen to let yourself go so far that you're bulging at the seams again, well, so what. It isn't worth cutting your throat about. You're not going to throw yourself off a cliff. You got it off once, you can get it off again. Maybe this time you'll learn something you missed before. Just claim temporary insanity and start over.

Don't forget to use your experience of miserably failing to keep the weight off to make you more understanding of others, who—through what you consider to be absolutely stupid behavior—mess up their lives. Remember that your inability to control your weight is perceived by some as a character flaw. While you and I know that's not true, others may not agree.

Anyway, regaining weight—after we promised ourselves faithfully, swore to the high heavens, that we'd never, never, never, be fat again—offers an unbeatable opportunity for learning to love. And after all, that's what we're here for.

Level Seven

"Thank You, Father. I Am Using That Thou Gavest Me."

In the meantime, now that you've got it, what do you do with it?

This thin body that you have worked for, sweated for, prayed for, must be good for something besides hanging pretty clothes on.

Is it enough to feel pride in your accomplishment? Will that keep you forever thin?

Is it enough not to be afraid to face your physician? Is his approval important enough to guarantee that you will never have to lose all that weight—again?

Probably not.

If you have transformed your body from fat to thin, you are a special person. You have developed discipline and insight not common to everyone. Your mind has expanded, your awareness level has risen. You're in a position to help. You can *give back*.

After losing their excess weight, Jean Nidech founded Weight Watchers; Lois Lindauer, Diet Workshop; Marcella Debs, Trim Clubs, Inc.; Esther Manz, TOPS; Roseanne (no last names permitted), Overeaters Anonymous.

Each of these women is giving as she has received.

But one doesn't have to become a professional in the weight-control field to be of service to others.

An equally effective way of giving back is by showing compassion to one who has yet to find the answer. Obesity is only one manifestation of destructive, compulsive behavior. It just so happens that obesity is more *visible* in most cases than alcoholism and drug addiction. But in any case, the act of praying for others who still suffer from self-abuse of any description—be it alcohol, drugs, or food—is not to be discounted as service to others.

Who can more sincerely intercede for others than we who have been there ourselves? Who can pray more earnestly from the heart for those who remain handicapped by their own lack of understanding than we who have come face to face with self?

When my sons were little boys, I took several harried ambulance rides to the hospital, so that even today an automatic response to a wailing siren is a compelling of spirit to *be there*, comforting, healing, clearing the way for the injured, the family, the doctors, and especially the ambulance driver. Surrounding the situation with Light assures the peaceful knowledge that spirit will be there for me if the need arises.

Likewise we can instantaneously pray, on the spot, for anyone with what we recognize as a need. That doesn't mean that every fat person needs prayer support. But it's easy to recognize the ones who do. Something in their eyes, reflecting our own memory of the pain we once felt, evokes a "please, God." At that moment the transference of love and hope is perceptible. It's something akin to when Jesus said, "I feel virtue go out of me."

If, as Cayce said, thoughts are things, this heartfelt response to another's need must necessarily be healing to the recipient as well as the giver. And that is no small thing.

Loving prayer for one another can never be pointless. We probably will never know how we affect others, but we can know that, as we plant the seeds of hope and love within another, we reap the harvest of hope and love within ourselves as our needs arise.

People helping people works. God has no feet but our feet, no mouth but our mouths, no mind but our minds with which to reach His children. He loves even those who wander aimlessly through lifetime after lifetime, seeking at-onement with Him through mazes of wild emotions and dead-end attitudes. And we can help. We can be an example to just one who may be blocked from the God within by an aspect of self that we have come to know from firsthand experience. Then we can truly say, "Thank You, Father. I am using that Thou gavest me."

THE EDGAR CAYCE LEGACIES

Among the vast resources which have grown out of the late Edgar Cayce's work are:

The Readings: Available for examination and study at the Association for Research and Enlightenment, Inc.,(A.R.E.®) at Virginia Beach, Va., are 14,256 readings consisting of 49,135 pages of verbatim psychic material plus related correspondence. The readings are the clairvoyant discourses given by Cayce while he was in a self-induced hypnotic sleep-state. These discourses were recorded in shorthand and then typed. Copious indexing and cross-indexing make the readings readily accessible for study.

Research and Information: Medical information which flowed through Cayce is being researched and applied by the research divisions of the Edgar Cayce Foundation. Work is also being done with dreams and other aspects of ESP. Much information is disseminated through the A.R.E. Press publications, *A.R.E. News* and *The A.R.E. Journal.* Coordination of a nationwide program of lectures and conferences is in the hands of the Department of Education. A library specializing in psychic literature is available to the public with books on loan to members. An extensive tape library has A.R.E. lectures available for purchase. Resource material has been made available for authors, resulting in the publication of scores of books, booklets and other material.

A.R.E. Study Groups: The Edgar Cayce material is most valuable when worked with in an A.R.E. Study Group, the text for which is *A Search for God,* Books I and II. These books are the outcome of eleven years of work by Edgar Cayce with the first A.R.E. group and represent the distillation of wisdom which flowed through him in the trance condition. Hundreds of A.R.E. groups flourish throughout the United States and other countries. Their primary purpose is to assist the members to know their relationship to their Creator and to become channels of love and service to others. The groups are nondenominational and avoid ritual and dogma. There are no dues or fees required to join a group although contributions may be accepted.

Membership: A.R.E. has an open-membership policy which offers attractive benefits.

For more information write A.R.E., Box 595, Virginia Beach, Va. 23451. To obtain information about publications, please direct your query to A.R.E. Press. To obtain information about joining or perhaps starting an A.R.E. Study Group, please direct your letter to the Study Group Department.